PART 1: THE PREPARATION

"Being deeply loved by someone gives you strength, while loving someone deeply gives you courage."

- Lao Tzu

CHAPTER 1: AND SO WE BEGIN

*"It took me quite a long time to develop a voice, and now that I
have it, I'm not going to be silent."*

- Madeleine Albright

As a private person I never planned to write about the hardest moment in my life. Sharing something so intimate. Being so vulnerable. The idea terrified me. But a desire to share a story to someday help others like myself, others with an unexpected birth story far outweighed my fear.

Growing up I always heard, 'when you're pregnant it's one foot in the grave and the other out'. That statement was a depressing contrast to how Hollywood glamourises it and how we women paint a pretty picture of birth, often not telling the full story. Looking back on it now, I realise the truth; births are life altering at best and traumatizing at worst.

Everyone pinpoints throwing up and sleepless nights, never highlighting the preparation involved. Focusing on the changes that redefine us physically, mentally, emotionally, spiritually and socially. No one advocates the importance of having support and how a lack of it could have ripple effects long after the baby is born.

I share my story to empower women around the world to initiate honest conversations. To reveal the essence of birth. To embrace the truth of it. To revisit how our ancestors gave birth and to challenge the practices we engage in today.

This book explores one of the most intimate times of my life so far, which I share to provide a voice to those who need it. To educate those reading about the pros and cons of home birth and explain why the hospital experience, just like the home birth experience, may not be for everyone. The point is to highlight there is no 'one size fits all' when it comes to birth and each person should be allowed the right to choose what's best for themselves.

My goal is not to say that one method is better than the other; rather, my desire is to expand our knowledge and way of thinking; to be open to and supportive of other ideas.

Gimme a Home Birth revisits the three parts of my birth journey: the preparation, the arrival and the moments after. Each part vital for my journey of self-healing and unveiling the silver lining after life throws an unexpected curveball. Part four opened the discussion to other mothers giving them a chance to have open conversation with each other and share parts of their stories. In the final part of the book, I give words of advice for mums and all involved in their support team.

I maintained the authenticity of my story and wrote it to the best of my ability based on my memory of what happened. In some cases, I also included a few points of view from my husband's side of the story.

A conscious effort was made to protect the innocent and a few names, locations and instances have been changed to protect their identities and organisations. My goal is to share my story but I won't throw anyone under the bus to do so.

It's an emotional journey that is still raw and fresh. As I wrote, I revisited that dark point in my life and became overcome with emotion. A time where I was angry, sad, hurt, lost and depressed. To come out of that dark place, sometimes the only thing that helped was to look down at my main reason for writing this book, my child curled up in that favourite position on one side, sucking a thumb.

Just seeing my little one reminds me of all the good parts of this journey. I remember my eager anticipation of getting pregnant, carrying my child for nine months and finally getting to hold that child in my arms and watch my baby grow. Never did I expect that the day we finally met, my whole life would change forever.

As a birth photographer, I couldn't help but yearn for what my own home birth would be like someday. Whenever anyone asked about my birth plan, I'd proudly state "Gimme a home birth any day." But home births even now are still somewhat taboo in Barbados and everyone had a negative opinion of what they thought home births were like. I saw birth as a time of peace, reflection and focus of bringing new life earth side, in a place I called home. A home birth for me represented a welcomed contrast to the horror stories I'd heard about the hospital and its high rate of caesarean sections, medications and unpleasant bedside manner. I never even considered the hospital as an option for me.

No harsh artificial lights, clinical scents, strange faces or anything unfamiliar. I wanted my birth to be as natural as possible without medication, in my own space with my midwife talking Alex and me through as I delivered our baby via water birth at home. I wanted to catch my baby and be the first to hold him or her in my arms and say, "Hello little one, your name is.... I'm your mummy and I love you."

Thinking back on all I had planned in comparison to the reality of what brought me here caused the tears I was holding back to stream down my face like a dam that finally broke free.

I'd been sitting for hours staring at the computer screen, unable to write, although I promised myself I would. As the rain started to fall, I smiled at the irony, as it was raining that day too, the day my baby was born. I walked to the window, using that memory to summon the strength I needed to write. Just the thought of writing scared me. Writing it all down meant I'd be reliving my experience all over again; the pain, the frustration, the anger, and the fear, the loneliness. Mainly the loneliness.

My thoughts were all over the place. What would people think? What would they say? Would they like it? Would they hate it? Did it even matter? I felt stuck. But this story was bigger than me. It was the beginning of a season of change; a way to let other mothers with a similar story know they're not alone. A way of bringing the reality of birth to the fore and equipping mothers-and fathers-to-be with the knowledge of their ability to choose another way if they so desire.

Taking a deep breath, I cleared my mind and mentally and emotionally returned to that day and the many moments leading up to it and all that brought me to the present. It was time…time to face my fears and share how I ended up with the birth story I didn't expect.

CHAPTER 2: LET'S MAKE A BABY

*"If you're offered a seat on a rocket ship, don't ask what seat!
Just get on."*

- Sheryl Sandberg

When you're married everyone asks when you're going to have a baby. But no one tells you how expensive it is, or how draining it is. No one discloses that your life as you know it will change forever. Having a baby was not a decision to be taken lightly. Alex and I had discussed this upfront and always wanted to wait about two years or so after we married before expanding our family.

Our lives were a little chaotic from inception. After getting married we started building a business and were preparing to build our own home. As newlyweds, we were still learning each other, as well as ourselves. Was there ever really a good time to add a little one to the mix? Fully aware of my maternal clock ticking, I didn't want to wait too late. My father often joked, saying I was no spring chicken, and Alex and I knew we didn't want to be fifty and running around behind a ten-year-old. But the cramped two-bedroom apartment, which doubled as our office space, just wasn't big enough. With one bedroom filled with lighting and photography equipment and the other as our actual bedroom, there just was no place for a nursery or anything else.

The more we talked about it, the more excited we became about being parents and having a baby. There was no perfect time anyway, right? We decided to start baby making in the New Year. We used condoms as our chosen form of contraception and I was curious to see what it would be like without them. I wasn't a big fan of any form of medication, so the pill was a definite no for me and there was no way I was having an intrauterine system or device installed.

With the decision made, I was full steam ahead looking at names for both boys and girls. Four of each, all beginning with the letter A, like Alex, and two middle names each, like me. Who knew that searching for names could be so much fun and so tedious? We spent hours researching the meanings of each name, as we wanted to choose names that reflected something positive. We ended up with a list of eight full possibilities ranging in meaning from 'beautiful maiden' to 'gift from God'.

Next, I started researching births, watching labour ward videos and reading as much as I could. It made me both scared and excited seeing those mums in labour. Some were screaming in pain, some had unexpected complications and others still made birth seem like a walk in the park.

Alex refused to watch any videos with me, but was intrigued by the idea of a home birth. I researched the pros and the cons of it, especially in comparison to the hospital, and reported my findings to Alex. We arranged a pre-consultation session with Tara, a certified midwife trained in the UK. I liked her almost immediately when I opened the door. She was tall, with gorgeous olive skin and an engaging smile. As she explained all to be considered for childbirth, her pleasant, gentle way of speaking confirmed in my mind that I was making the right decision. Tara guided us on how to go about preparing on each core level – mental, physical, emotional and spiritual. She impressed me with her knowledge and patience in answering my many questions.

She highlighted the importance of diet, nutrition and exercise, explaining how anything we did now could positively or negatively impact our birth. She gave us a lot of literature and asked us to begin to visualise our birth from now, even down to the energy in the birthing area. Tara promoted the sacred nature of the birth space, stressing how easy it was for any negative energy to affect it. I had no idea that preparing for a baby was such an involved process and wondered how many people actually went through the same preparation.

With twins running on both sides of our family, I was silently hoping for two bundles of joy, much to Alex's dismay. He was of the strong opinion that juggling one baby at any time would be enough to have our hands full.

Eager to start the preparation, we opted to do the fourteen-day detox Tara recommended. Now take my advice if you've never done a fourteen-day detox, or any detox for that matter, it's something you want to give some serious thought to first. Let me tell you, it wasn't easy. More like brutal. No sugars, no dairy, no chicken or fish, no processed anything. No food as far as I was concerned. Don't get me wrong I wouldn't say we were terrible eaters but working a nine to five and building a business together didn't help with eating habits. We spent a lot of time on the road, rushing from here to there, so fast food became a major convenience. This detox was definitely like going cold turkey, especially for Alex who had a sweet tooth and craved anything with milk.

Discussing a meal plan beforehand would have helped significantly. I didn't do one and was scrambling daily to find something to survive on, which often led to hunger and frustration. I felt overwhelmed trying to decide what to eat. I was not a fan of vegetables. I proudly maintained a limited intake of coleslaw, tomatoes and lettuce on a burger, which I truly believed were vegetables enough.

Eventually, with a few salads and a bit of cheese in between, we made it to the thirteenth day. My small frame gave the appearance of hard times and my once tight-fitting clothes hung a bit too loose in some pertinent areas of my anatomy. Alex wasn't complaining too much as somehow, in spite of the weight loss, we had gained a bunch of energy from cutting out the excess crap from our regular diets. Day thirteen, though, was rough. We had just covered a four-hour photography event and were both tired and more than a bit cranky. As we turned to leave, the organiser invited us to have something to eat. After a quick exchange, Alex and I bid farewell to the detox, as the offer of food was too tempting to refuse.

With the detox out of the way, the next step was to find a suitable OB/GYN to get a check-up. I wasn't a fan of doctors and needed to find the right person for the job. He or she had a critical role to play. After much deliberation and a few recommendations from Tara, we eventually settled on Melissa Knowles, a lady with a great track record for her professionalism and experience in the field. We scheduled an appointment with her and were quite happy when she gave me a clean bill of health.

Months had passed and we'd researched as much as anyone could to get ourselves ready to have a baby. But something was still holding us back. Were we sure we were ready? Was I ready? Would I ever really be? One thing I knew for sure was I wasn't getting any younger and I was tired waiting. Tired of second guessing myself. I knew everything wasn't in order, but I couldn't shake this desire to be a mummy. I wanted a baby.

It was mid-December and the Christmas chill was in the air. Alex was fast asleep. I listened to his light snore as I lay awake wrestling with the rationale of if now was the best time to be a mum. I couldn't take it anymore. I reached over and whispered into his ear, "Let's make a baby." Smiling and with lightning speed, Alex rolled on top of me with mischief dancing in his eyes and said, "It's about time." It was the first time we'd be getting to know each other without protection. It felt good, so we tried and tried again.

CHAPTER 3: I'M PREGNANT

"What we have once enjoyed we can never lose. All that we love deeply becomes a part of us."

- Helen Keller

Christmas came and went and the New Year was in full swing. We had a number of photography events to cover so my focus was on getting the work done. The jobs were mounting and Alex also had a bunch of graphic designs to complete but something wasn't right. Somehow, I just couldn't sleep. I felt heavy and bloated and somehow my chest seemed like it weighed a ton. What was going on? I hoped I hadn't overworked myself and was now coming down with something.

By mid-February, I was exhausted and still wasn't sleeping well. Lying on my back was almost painful and lying on my stomach made me feel like my breasts would explode. Alex suggested I call Tara, so I did. Immediately after describing my symptoms, she suggested I take a pregnancy test. With all that was going on the thought hadn't even crossed my mind and I made a mental note not to get excited just in case it was a false alarm. I picked up the phone again, this time to call a friend of mine that I often referred to as 'The Veteran'. She had three babies and was expecting her fourth any day now and she was still sane, so yes, she was a veteran indeed. I told her what was happening and she, too, suggested I take a pregnancy test. The next day Alex and I went out and bought one.

Could I be pregnant already? Only then did I realise that my period was late and it usually comes like clockwork. Could it be? Out of nowhere a bunch of butterflies escaped and flew circles around my belly. Alex laughed as I went through my rollercoaster of emotions, from happy to scared to everything in between. After a while, he urged me to just relax and pee on the stick and so I did, careful to follow all the instructions on the package. We waited for what seemed like an hour but was probably only five minutes before we saw that second purple line appear on the stick. I consulted the box to confirm what the two lines meant. I looked at Alex, who was smiling back at me and I couldn't contain my emotions any longer. It was positive. "AhhHHHH!" I screamed and danced in excitement before he shushed me. "We're going to have a baby," I said and screamed again. He only laughed and pulled me in for a hug before reminding me not to talk too loudly and be overheard by the neighbours.

We knew the risks of pregnancy and how vulnerable babies are, especially in the first trimester, and we promised not to say anything to anyone until we had reached the thirteen-week mark. It felt like so much fun to keep our little secret to ourselves. Two days later, Tara invited us to a session with her charity group comprising of a number of persons who supported and encouraged home births. After the session, one of the members there turned to us and said congratulations. Glancing quickly at Alex, I said thank you and hurriedly made an exit. When I got to the car, Alex said, "I wonder what made him say that" "I haven't a clue," was all I could say as I smiled down, rubbing my tummy.

My boobs were growing, much to my surprise and Alex's delight. Even my sister said I was looking rosy and all I could do was smile. But as the days wore on, I started to notice little spots of blood and immediately called Tara. She assured me it was nothing to worry about but to keep her posted if anything changed. Sure enough, later that week, everything changed.

As colleagues of mine strolled into the office, I was already typing away, eager to send off some emails before I moved on to the rest of my tasks when a sharp pain started in the pit of my stomach. Thinking I needed to eat, I took out a snack and repositioned myself in the chair in hopes of easing my discomfort. When Alex called five minutes later to discuss the possibility of covering a wedding photography request in our schedule, I told him about the pain. He, as usual, suggested I call Tara if the discomfort persisted and we continued to analyse the schedule. There was no way we could cover this wedding with everything else we had to do that weekend. Before I ended the call, I promised to contact the potential client and let them know we were unavailable.

The discomfort in my stomach continued and I fought the urge to cry out in pain. No one at work knew I was pregnant yet and I wanted to keep it that way, not just because I was still only five weeks in, but also because I didn't trust the people I worked with. As I scanned the room, I made a quick decision to walk to the washroom while Cheryl, the chief instigator and busybody, was still distracted on the phone. Cheryl was the mover and shaker in the office, always in the know and in the do. She made it her business to get into everyone's business and had this way of staring at me that made me very uncomfortable. I was grateful for the job. It paid the bills. But the environment, both physically and emotionally, left much to be desired.

I walked to the bathroom, grateful as the discomfort began to subside, and gave my tummy a gentle rub. I was looking forward to mummyhood and watching my tummy grow. I squatted above the toilet bowl to relieve my bladder and looked down to see a red ball on my underwear. It was only then that I understood the source of the pain and water rolled freely down my cheeks as I stared at that ball that told the story of the life I'd just lost.

Gingerly removing the small red ball and managing to relieve my swollen bladder, another ball fell into the bowl. I never knew that my heart could sink further. Barely composing myself, I returned to my desk, grabbed my phone and rushed outside to an open space. I needed to breathe. I needed some air. I could feel the panic rising in me as my brain tried to catch up with everything I was feeling. I had to remind myself to hold it together but when I finally called Alex to tell him what had happened everything I was holding in was unleashed and I broke down and cried right there in the open. I cried for the child I never knew. The child that only Alex and I knew existed. I cried for the life that was now lost. No longer able to stand, I fell to my knees as the blame fell upon me and nothing Alex said could console me. I stayed outside long after we hung up before I returned to my desk, grabbed my bags and left. Cheryl muttered something about how people don't tell you where they're going, but I didn't care. I needed to be home and far away from this place.

As I left to head home, all I could think of was what had happened in the bathroom at work. Maybe I was overreacting and it wasn't what I thought it was. Still holding a sliver of hope, I grabbed the last pregnancy test as soon as I got in the house and waited impatiently for the two lines to once again appear. But the two lines never showed. The test was negative and my baby was gone. I walked over, lay on the bed and cried well into the night.

I spent the next few weeks blaming myself. My mind went through a cycle of if only I had eaten properly, if only I wasn't stressing so much at work, if only I didn't suddenly change my diet, maybe if I went to bed earlier. Alex didn't know what to do or what to say, which left me feeling lonelier than ever. I couldn't talk to anyone else about it, so I comforted myself with Google articles and support groups which helped me to come to terms with what they described as early miscarriage, a pregnancy loss before ten weeks. It helped to know I wasn't alone.

When I was finally up for it, we scheduled an appointment with Melissa, the OB/GYN, to give me a check-up. She listened as I explained my loss, but she, too, didn't seem to understand how devastated I really felt. Maybe I'd just imagined the whole thing, but as my body returned to what it was before and my boobs shrank back to regular size, I knew it was true. No matter what Melissa or Alex said, I knew what had happened and my baby was gone.

It took me a while to mentally prepare for baby making again. I was scared to get excited again. I was scared to get pregnant and then have to face the possibility of losing another baby. I didn't know what to do, but Alex was patient and encouraging and coaxed me into it.

Baby making was a fun exercise and it definitely called for some creativity. During the day and during the night, we learned how to make each session more enjoyable than the last. But part of me was holding back. I was still scared. I didn't want to lose another life. No matter how early that life was or how short I knew that life existed, it was a new life within me.

Alex picked up on my vibe. Somehow, he sensed it and that night he made it his business to assure me that everything would be okay. His words and all he did reminded me of his love for me, and my love for him. In that moment, I knew another life was being conceived and we'd just made a baby. I looked into his gleaming brown eyes as he lay breathing heavily and I knew that he knew as well.

CHAPTER 4: EVERYBODY HAS SOMETHING TO SAY

"The woman who does not require validation from anyone is the most feared individual on the planet."

- Mohadesa Najumi

I was pregnant again and starting to show. Every day that he or she got stronger, I was grateful. Grateful and excited to eventually see that tiny face and to hold my child in my arms. I was enjoying the journey. I even enjoyed the two weeks of morning sickness where all that would stay down was apples… and I hated apples.

When we made it past the thirteen-week mark, we gave our parents the good news. We showed up to our parents' homes, handed our mums a small glass baby bottle and said, "When you travel, buy glass." It took a while for them to get it, but when they finally did, they were over the moon. It'd be my parents' first grandchild and Alex's parents' second. My mum was already making plans of what she'd buy for the baby and all the trips they'd take, but all I wanted was for this baby to be happy, healthy and whole.

Everyone wanted to know the gender of the baby, but I didn't want to and Alex was fine with my decision. To me, that was part of what made it so special, the not knowing until he or she was born. I loved the mystery and excitement of it. To ensure no one spilled the beans, I told Melissa up front not to tell us if she made any discoveries during the ultrasound. My mother complained a bit about not knowing what clothes to buy, but I told her the same as I told everyone else buy neutral colours, yellow, white and green. The gender didn't matter because his or her name was ready for when he or she arrived.

The more people found out, the more real it all felt. And it didn't cease to amaze me how some people gave their opinions when they were never asked for or even desired. Everybody had an opinion. Everybody had something to say. Friends. Family. Co-workers. Strangers. Most of the time I just found it annoying. It ranged from the food I ate to the shoes I wore to when I could wash my hair. I know in most instances they meant well, but I felt bombarded with so many persons all at once.

I was just over six months pregnant and each week it seemed like I gained another ten pounds. I was still getting used to my swollen abdomen and shrinking bladder and was so appreciative of this tiny human growing inside me. But I felt as big as a bus. And it didn't help that the comfortable pants I wanted to wear on Monday wouldn't fit, although I wore them just the Thursday prior.

Thankfully there were a few of us who were pregnant around the same time, so it helped to have others to exchange pregnancy tales of swollen feet and unsolicited belly rubs. It was a playful exchange of wardrobe wars and a new understanding of bladder care. We created a game to reveal which businesses were kind enough to allow us to use their washrooms. Not all of them were and it was almost like a treasure hunt to find out that these washrooms even exist. We encouraged each other on our down days, when doubts or fears arose. It was great to have others to talk to about baby items. It was only when I got pregnant that I realised how little information I really had on pregnancy and birth.

Everyone knows that babies usually come around nine months after conception, but once you're pregnant your care providers count everything in weeks. This in itself was enough to drive me crazy. I could never remember, but somehow Alex always seemed to get it right.

Pregnancy hunger was another thing to get used to. The hunger was real. Tara always reminded me I wasn't eating for two like people often suggest, but I was definitely eating more and needed to be mindful of my vitamin and mineral intake. Too little or too much could impact baby with things like spina bifida, when the spine and spinal cord don't properly form as a possible result of folate deficiency.

I had no clue that expectant mothers were required to have so many tests done. Glucose tests, Down Syndrome tests, urine tests, blood tests and ultrasounds. I drew the line at someone sticking a needle in my unborn baby's spine though. Everything was about checking just in case something was wrong, but my baby was fine and I was not exposing him or her to a host of unnecessary tests.

Working in the middle of the hustle and bustle, I was very reluctant to venture outside. Somehow, a pregnant belly seemed to bring out the absolute extremes in people and I was afraid of random people touching my belly. At first, I thought I was just being paranoid, but one day while photographing an event, another photographer whom Alex and I were familiar with suddenly reached out and rubbed my tummy, wished me well and walked away. I restrained the urge to hit him with the camera. Alex wasn't pleased at all about what happened and made a note to be more vigilant. This was the first of many in a series of unsolicited events.

While walking through the mall two days later, a former work colleague rounded the corner and, noticing my pregnant belly, rushed forward ready to touch. Instinctively, I grabbed her hands and pushed them away from my unborn child. She looked at me with what looked like a mixture of shock and disbelief, which only annoyed me. But the icing on the cake was when she asked if I don't like people touching my belly. When I said no, she said, "But it's a rite of passage." People never used to touch my stomach before I was pregnant and that wasn't going to change. It's my personal space and it didn't matter what she or anyone else thought.

Being pregnant, though enjoyable, was exhausting. I felt the need to constantly protect myself by placing a bag or a book in front of my belly. Not only did I have to be physically ready but I had to be mentally ready as well.

At work, Cheryl and her clique decided it best to share their personal horror stories of birth whenever I was around, trying anything to get a rise out of me. This was a whole new level of wickedness on their part, done in spite because I didn't share any information with them about my pregnancy. But I vowed not to let it affect me.

One particular day I'd had enough of these stories about miscarriage and birth complications and decided that anytime the conversations went that way, I'd simply leave the room. Knowing what I'd already suffered while working in this place and the life I already lost there, I didn't want anything negative to impact this new life that was growing. Maybe they caught the drift, maybe they didn't, but I no longer cared. My number one priority was creating a healthy environment for my unborn child and this workplace only proved time and time again that this wasn't it.

Both Tara and Alex wanted me to take at least two weeks to centre myself before the baby was born, but I wanted to work right up. I just didn't want to cut my time with baby short. I was saving up my vacation days wherever possible so I could add them to the end of my maternity leave. It annoyed me to think I was expected to grow a tiny human for nine months and then only spend a quarter of the year with him or her before I'm expected to return to work. That's crazy. Even exclusive breastfeeding was suggested for six months. So, I didn't want to waste a day.

After a while Cheryl and her group started to wear on my resolve and were becoming unbearable, and the general negativity of the work environment was weighing heavily on me. I didn't welcome the horror stories nor the alternate days of interrogation that followed. Persons decided to ask about where we were having the baby. Which hospital? How far along are you? What sex is the baby? And as usual, the constant glares. Even Sarah, who used to be a close friend back in the day, was in on the stares, but she dared not ask. We weren't friends anymore and I doubted we'd ever be again.

CHAPTER 5: WE'RE HAVING A HOME BIRTH

"Words are, of course, the most powerful of medicine used by mankind."

- Rudyard Kipling

We disclosed to a few persons that we were having a home birth and I regretted that decision almost immediately. I remember the day I first told my parents. My mother's response was priceless. She stated everything from the risks to the fact that that's what people used to do back in the day. She felt it was unsafe and basically an unnecessary thing to do in this day and age. It felt as if every day she found yet another reason why I should go to the hospital.

My dad, who isn't very outspoken unless really upset or behind a pulpit, remained quiet during the exchange, but I could tell that he, too, didn't approve of the idea. Of the two, he was always more accepting of me and my outside-the-norm decisions. But I could see his hesitation and reluctance as Alex took the time to carefully explain our birth plan. He asked a few questions here and there and seemed contented enough that we did have a backup plan in place just in case anything was to go wrong. But it bothered me that we didn't have his full support.

My brother on the other hand, in his usual colourful way, simply replied, "Them does still do that? Ok, so then after you go to the hospital?" I almost laughed but I knew he was just genuinely concerned; they all were. But so was I. Concerned that no one seemed to care about the simple fact that it was my decision. As the mother of my unborn child, I had final say in what I thought was best.

As time wore on, we explained to our parents the role Tara would play in everything. We discussed her overall requirements and procedures and her disclaimer that she would only be able to provide her service once my pregnancy remained low-risk. If the baby didn't arrive before forty-two weeks or if I developed preeclampsia, high blood pressure during pregnancy or any other life-threatening birth complication, she would, by law, have to refer me to the hospital as she was not a doctor and we'd need to get to one immediately should trouble arise.

We relayed the same information to Alex's parents, who gave a similar reaction. I could tell that they, too, were concerned. Everyone wanted to know about the what-ifs. What if something went wrong? What if your emergency driver doesn't get there in time? They were always sure to ask: "Are you sure this is what you want?" I was sure. It was what I wanted more than anything. I wanted to give birth in my own home, in a place I was familiar with and gave me the freedom to move around as I saw fit. I didn't want to be under those harsh bright lights and surrounded by all those hospital smells while lying in an unfamiliar bed. I wanted to be home with Alex.

Since photographing my first home birth a few years prior and seeing the true beauty of birth in its most natural form, there was no way I was going to do anything else. I was able to witness it first-hand and longed to have the same strength and power my client displayed when I birthed a child of my own. I spent hours talking with the midwives there about the entire process and fell in love with the concept. This was the right decision for me.

Not wanting any parents in the room also sparked another discussion. I guess Alex's parents expected it, but my mum was surprised and I guess hurt that I didn't want her there. Don't get me wrong, I love my mum terribly, but I needed peace and quiet and strength in my birth space. I needed persons who were fully supportive of our decision and my mum just wasn't. So, I only wanted Alex in that space along with my birth team, Tara, my midwife, and Sheena, my doula. As a doula, Sheena was trained to provide guidance and support during labour and help maintain my focus and remind me of what I was fighting for and what my body was capable of. I wanted no negativity in the birth space.

My mum wanted to be there to see the birth of her first grandchild. She was excited and a part of me wanted her there, but I knew it was for the best if she wasn't. I could see she was disappointed and more than a little hurt but both Alex and I agreed and I wasn't about to change my mind. I knew my mum had mentioned it to my dad the minute he brought it up one day when he was driving me home. He was trying to get me to understand it from my mother's point of view and highlighted how important something like this was for her and how happy she'd be to see the birth. He didn't want me to take the moment away from her and suggested that I could let her stay for a couple hours.

Listening to my father only confirmed why I shouldn't change my mind. This wasn't about my mother; it was about me, Alex and our baby and trusting God that everything would be all right. How happy she'd be?!? What about me? This was my first baby, and Alex and I wanted to ensure we had the right supportive energy around us to create a safe space for our son or daughter to enter the world.

Little did I know that this lack of support for our home birth and the stress from work had already started to plant seeds of doubt in my subconsciousness. Doubt that would later make its presence known and felt.

As the due date approached, we made a special effort to get all the items Tara had on the list, including incontinence sheets (padded sheets to contain any involuntary bodily fluids), old towels, oxytocin and a designated driver in case of an emergency hospital transfer. She also recommended that we purchase a birthing kit and ensure that we had an oxygen cylinder on hand, equipped with an adapter, regulator and key, along with a baby-sized oxygen mask.

I alternated between Tara and Melissa for my antenatal check-ups. During each session they examined the baby, took my weight and blood pressure and educated me on maintaining exercise and a well-balanced diet. Each session was interesting and pleasant but I wasn't a fan of being poked and prodded.

Tara also insisted that I still go to the local hospital for an antenatal check-up, just to be sure they had paperwork for me. I was reluctant at first and even a little upset by her suggestion, but she assured me that it was only to ensure that all of our bases were covered. The reality was that with birth we had no control. It could go well or it could go badly and if things got hazy in any way Tara wanted to ensure that if there was any need for a sudden hospital transfer, nothing would delay my admittance.

Reluctantly, two weeks before the baby was due, Alex and I walked into the hospital and sat in the waiting room. I was not looking forward to this visit and my anxiety was showing. I hated the hospital and had a slight thing against doctors and nurses. I comforted myself that this was only a quick check-up to get my name in the system and that was it.

The small room was packed with people of all ages. We said good morning and walked to the front desk only to be asked by a visibly annoyed nurse if we had read the sign. Before I could ask her what she meant, she pointed to a handwritten sign, which stated to pull a number and have a seat. Working hard not to get aggravated, I pulled a number and we took the last remaining seats. I was grateful that Alex hadn't listened to me and had taken the time off to be here. Most of the other mums were sitting by themselves.

We'd been waiting for at least an hour before the nurse rounded us up like a herd to go and pee in a cup and get our pressure checked. There was no paper in the bathroom and I wondered for the hundredth time why I was even here in this place.

When I was finally called in for the check-up, a trainee doctor greeted me with long talons for nails. She handed me a sheet of flipchart paper and asked me to place it on the bed and lie on it after I got undressed. I looked at the bed and tried not to let my mind get carried away. As far as doctors go, she was pleasant enough, but as she explored my swollen belly, I held my tongue rather than express how uncomfortable her nails were. She went through the routine quickly and got the senior physician, who didn't even bat an eyelash in my direction, to sign off. I remember thinking it's just this one visit and praying that was true.

As the days wore on, it was getting harder and harder to visualise my ideal birth. There was still so much to do in terms of preparing the house and getting all the necessary baby supplies. I was beginning to feel overwhelmed. Going to work didn't help much as Cheryl and her crew continued to play their games and tell tales of births gone wrong. I could tell she was very upset that I didn't tell her I was pregnant, but I was showing so she could see for herself.

I started to get thoughts of things going wrong and felt a sense of fear rising in the pit of my stomach. With more than enough on my plate, it didn't help when my father told me that the head of the antenatal unit had said that home births were illegal and suggested that I get to the nearest hospital when my labour was underway. Illegal? Could that really be true? How could it be illegal for me to birth my child at home? I started to Google it, searching every article I could find, but nothing supported her claim. What she said was ignorant at best and utterly disgusting at worst and I was disturbed and disappointed that my father had even bothered to share her statement with me in the first place. That really was something he could've kept to himself.

Defending my birth decision was exhausting and it was starting to wear me down. As I reached down and rubbed my swollen belly, I wondered if things like this were said to other women. I wondered if they, too, got scared after hearing tales of what could go wrong. I knew I was. Just days earlier, an elderly lady was talking to me and thought it necessary to share her opinion of birth and how glad she was we had hospitals now to reduce the number of deaths they used to have back in the day when people gave birth at home.

I wanted a home birth. I wanted to have a pool filled with water in the middle of our house and to have my favourite music playing to set the mood. I wanted to be the one to catch my baby. To pull him or her out of the water and say the child's name. To look Alex in his eyes and say, "Hello, daddy." I wanted a delayed cutting of the cord or for the cord to be burnt if we could and to bury my placenta in the yard. Then I wanted to rest, just the three of us as the midwife and doula left. To enjoy the moments of the day Alex and I became parents and thank God for the miracle he allowed us to perform.

CHAPTER 6: I DON'T FEEL SO GOOD

*"I learned from my mother that there is a greatness in all of us,
and that all of us are delivered to this world with a mission."*

- Les Brown

The countdown was on. At thirty-eight weeks pregnant, I was definitely larger than I'd ever been in my life, weighing a hefty hundred and fifty-five pounds and round. Very round. I was excited. I was scared. I was a bundle of mixed emotions.

I planned on working right up until the baby was due, but Tara and Alex insisted that I take some time off to mentally prepare myself for the next step of this journey – the delivery. Eventually I gave in and sent in my request to get one week off. Jennifer, my supervisor and the only one in the office I had trusted enough to tell I was pregnant, was relieved that I was taking the time. She was aware of my daily struggles and oftentimes provided a listening ear when I needed to vent about Cheryl or any of my colleagues. She also made me feel valued, like what I did mattered. Jennifer was a rare gem that I greatly appreciated in an otherwise depressing work environment.

Even with Jennifer's support, work continued to be a struggle, as my colleagues didn't take well to my 'keep to myself' routine. As usual, Cheryl had much to say, often launching into lengthy discussions about how back in the day they used to be a team but now that had all changed and people don't talk to each other like before. She always said the same thing over and over again to anyone who would listen, leaving me to resort to the comfort of my headphones and my music.

She spoke of 'team' as though it were oxygen, but I had never met such selfish people, each looking to get ahead of the other, maintaining great levels of pretence, smiling in your face and crucifying you behind your back. Many went out of their way to inquire about my pregnancy but some were just content to stare. Neither was welcomed and I was eagerly looking forward to my time away.

Although Sarah and I used to be close friends years ago, the minute I started to work here she decided to treat me like dirt, not willing to show me where the lunchroom was or to bring me a chair from upstairs after mine was broken. Sarah got upset when I got married and had been holding a grudge ever since. Her actions really hurt me especially seeing as she was the one that encouraged me to come and work here in the first place. Many nights I went home in tears telling Alex about how she treated me that day, and things she said behind my back that she thought I never knew. I figured if she, someone who knew me for years, even before I came to work at this place, could treat me as badly as that, everyone else could, so I kept to myself.

It was approaching midday when the familiar urge to pee started to awaken my bladder for what felt like the hundredth time that day. Waddling down the hall, a sharp pain pierced my stomach and I fought the urge to cry out. Moving as fast as my legs would allow, I made it to the bathroom and leaned against the wall. I tried hard not to worry as the still vivid memory of the last time I had such a pain threatened my resolve. Gently rubbing my belly, I said a silent prayer that all would be well. I didn't want to lose this child. Lord knew I couldn't handle it; not now. Not so close to meeting him or her.

After the pain passed, I returned to my desk. Alex always teased me saying that he could tell I was trying to move my legs fast but I still wasn't going anywhere. I could see him laughing at me now as I sat and the chair squeaked under the weight.

Settled in my seat, my little one started kicking up a storm. That had to be a good sign, right? I hoped so. I thought of messaging Alex but decided against it. I wouldn't. Not yet. The discomfort reminded me of menstrual cramps, but with a bit more of something else that I wasn't quite sure how to explain. After some time passed, I finally called Alex just to give him an update. He assured me that all would be fine, but asked me to keep monitoring it and to call Tara if anything changed.

As the day progressed, so did the discomfort. It was becoming more and more difficult to sit still. I needed to readjust in an effort to get more comfortable. I was also painfully aware of Cheryl and her eagle eyes that kept scanning over me. At least she wasn't sharing any traumatic birth stories today and for the most part was keeping her mouth shut.

By midday I still wasn't feeling any better and was desperate to lie down. As I turned to head out to lunch, Cheryl surprised me by asking when I was going on leave. Smiling, I opened the door and simply said not yet. I still had one more week before I took my vacation and two more weeks before my expected delivery. Looking down at my stomach as baby started kicking again, I wondered if this little one was giving me a sign of other plans.

I could hardly eat anything and decided maybe I should leave work early after all. Alex had a funeral to attend and insisted I come so he could take me straight home after. I told Jennifer that I would leave early and she agreed, so I logged off my workstation and packed up my stuff to go.

Who would have thought that just being away from the office would help. I remember thinking that I really should have listened to Tara and taken the two weeks off, but it was too late for that now.

The funeral was surprisingly cheerful and it had a calmness to it that was comforting. I was still experiencing the discomfort though, and appreciated when the minister wrapped up his message so we could head home.

Alex helped me to the van and I could see the concern on his face, as I could no longer hide the discomfort etched on mine. I tried to assure him that all was well, hoping he believed it, although I was having a hard time believing it myself. I was tired and just prayed that nothing was wrong with our baby. I didn't care about the gender. I just wanted a baby who was of sound mind and in good health with everything intact. A baby that was happy, healthy and whole and I wanted to be here to meet him or her.

As soon as we got home I headed to the shower before finally climbing into bed, but that didn't offer as much relief as I'd thought. I was tossing and turning, finding it hard to locate that sweet spot. I tried lying on my left side as I'd read this helps with blood flow for the baby, but for some reason I just couldn't get comfortable. Alex came and asked if I was sure that I didn't want to call Tara, but I really didn't want to bother her. Besides, my parents were coming back from their travels and I wanted to go to the airport to welcome them back. I knew if I didn't go my mum would worry. She was getting anxious about seeing her first grandchild and was being overly protective of us both. It felt good to be fussed over sometimes.

We got to the airport just after 7:30 p.m. and had to wait for my parents to clear customs. I was not doing too well and those hard airport benches did nothing to offer relief. However, they were still better than standing on my now swollen ankles. Just the week before I was telling someone that at least I didn't get swollen feet and now look. The irony of it. I spotted my parents coming and, as I stood, I all but winced in pain. Daddy seemed oblivious to my discomfort, but mummy, who sometimes moved like she had the eyes of a hawk, squinted at me, taking it all in.

By the time we got home and I had to walk up the driveway, I could sense rather than see my mother analysing my every move. She knew something was up but didn't ask, so I didn't tell. Maybe I should have stayed home after all. I avoided eye contact, making a mental note to walk as straight as I could. I didn't want them to worry, I just needed some rest and I'd be good. I hoped.

PART 2: THE BIRTH

"Never apologise for being sensitive or emotional. Let this be a sign that you've got a big heart and aren't afraid to let others see it. Showing your emotions is a sign of strength."

- Brigitte Nicole

CHAPTER 7: IT'S TIME

"The greatest mistake you can make in life is to be continually fearing you will make one."

- Elbert Hubbard

I woke up the next day, tired, groggy and in pain. I'd been tossing and turning the whole night, trying my best to get comfortable and not wake Alex. There was no way I'd make it to work today.

The pain had intensified and my back felt like it was on fire. Nothing I did seemed to be outing the growing flames. It was around 7:00 a.m. and Alex wanted me to call Tara, but I was reluctant. Realising the pain was getting worse, he went ahead and called her anyway and she just confirmed what I was already starting to think. It was time. The baby was coming. My heart and my head were in conflict. I wanted to see my child, but I wasn't ready. The nursery wasn't done, my emergency bag wasn't packed, and mentally I was exhausted. We'd only just managed to put up the crib, changer and dresser that were bought for us. I still had two more weeks.

I was starting to panic, but before I had a chance to get more carried away in my thoughts, I felt another contraction, one that nearly brought me to my knees. My back was on fire. Okay, this was no longer feeling like menstrual pain. After another hour of five-minute intervals of pain, I whispered for Alex to tell Tara to come. She said it was still early as first-time mums usually take a while to deliver but I wanted her here now. I was getting scared.

Alex left soon after the call. He went over to his dad's house to get some large pots and pans to help boil the water to fill the pool. He also called my dad who headed off to the hospital to collect my paperwork. My mum was getting anxious and kept calling to ask if she could come, but I said no. Her nervous energy was making me even more nervous.

Tara came shortly after and confirmed that I was still in what was considered to be the latent or early phase of labour and encouraged me to breathe and walk around if I needed to. She was calm and relaxed and that helped me to focus and remain at ease. The assisting midwife and Sheena, the doula, both arrived an hour later. The presence of so many persons surprisingly started to make me nervous. It was only three people, but it felt like twenty and I wasn't used to so many people in the house.

I was having second thoughts. Maybe I should have just had Tara, but there was nothing I could do to change neither that nor my regret for not renting the TENS machine - a transcutaneous electrical nerve stimulation machine offering a non-invasive method of providing pain relief. Everything was becoming very costly so I had told Alex the machine wasn't necessary, but the intensifying pain in my back was a constant reminder that I'd made a bad decision.

I knew I needed to focus on the task at hand of safely delivering this baby into the world, but I felt tired, depressed and unprepared. I fought the wave of negative thoughts that were swirling around in my head, instead focusing on Tara, Alex and the others boiling water to fill the birth pool. My baby was on the way. I smiled at the thought of holding my little one in my arms that same night.

Tara encouraged me to move around, eat and just relax as best I could. After all, I was home and could pretty much do what I pleased. Knowing I'd be getting hungry, Alex left to get everyone pizza. We forgot to get groceries this weekend and I was in no position to cook anything. When Alex returned, I wolfed down about four slices along with Tara's fruit salad. I was happy that I could eat and grateful for her reminders to drink juice and water to stay hydrated. Giving birth was like running a marathon, not a sprint and Tara was of the opinion that eating and drinking helped to maintain energy levels. The hospitals prohibit eating once admitted and that was another reason I was glad to be home.

Time seemed to be standing still. As the contractions intensified it became difficult to remember Tara's breathing techniques. The baby was pressing even harder on my bladder, making passing water more frequent and more difficult with the growing bonfire at the base of my spine. I remember one moment in particular being frozen on the toilet seat from the pain with tears cascading down my cheeks. Tara called Alex away from the pool to sit with me and I welcomed the quiet of just the two of us.

Alex reminded me of how powerful I was, and that I could do this and bring our baby here safely. I fought the urge to yell, "But you're not the one with a bonfire in your back and a basketball now about to force its way through your vagina!" I knew he meant well. I knew he did, but I wanted more than just words. I wanted him beside me in the water with me, just holding me. But he had a habit of being a bit distant and hands off at the most critical times.

I needed to have periodic vaginal exams. I hated them. They were uncomfortable, but I knew Tara was just checking to see how I was progressing. I was still only four centimetres and getting more and more tired and worried. A number of hours had passed but I seemed stuck somehow at four centimetres with no obvious signs of progression. I was losing my resolve as the what-ifs came out in full battle mode to flood my mind with doubts. But I fought to regain control.

Seemingly sensing my mental war, Tara pulled Alex and me into the bedroom. She wanted me to clear my mind of any inhibitive thoughts because she was concerned that something was holding me back. As soon as she turned to go, I told Alex how scared I was and what was swirling around in my head. Things from my past, the negative opinions friends and family shared and even those from work came to mind. It felt like I was sinking into quicksand, and the more I struggled, the deeper I sank. Alex held me close and gave me a moment to just release it all. After a few more minutes, I lifted my head off his shoulder and dried my tears. I was ready to give my all.

Alex YouTubed some of my favourite motivational speakers: Eric Thomas and Les Brown. I could feel the synergy in the room change and felt a new surge of energy to move forward. Tara showed Alex how to apply pressure to my back to ease the pain and how to assist me in using his exercise bar to do deep squats to relieve the pressure in my pelvic area. It was heading into late evening and the sun had already started to retire for the night but I was still at four centimetres. Nothing seemed to be working to bring this baby down and my energy was dwindling as I became more physically and mentally exhausted.

I lay in the birth pool feeling helpless but silently praying for my baby to arrive. It was almost 7:00 p.m. and Tara wanted me to consider transferring to the hospital, as I still was not dilating further. I begged for another hour or two, not wanting to give up but feeling somewhere inside me that the home birth I so longed for was now out of arm's reach.

The pool offered comfort, helping me to get a few naps between contractions and soothe the pain. I opened my eyes and glanced at the time. It was almost 9:00 p.m. Time was up. I turned to see that Alex and Tara were sitting on the couch with similar looks on their faces. Something was definitely wrong. The OB/GYN's office had called. The results were back. I had a positive test for Group B Strep. My heart sank. Group B Strep, though relatively harmless to adults, can cause babies to be critically ill with symptoms ranging from irritability to fever, meningitis or pneumonia.

Both the OB/GYN and a paediatrician whom Tara often partnered with recommended I take an oral antibiotic as baby's first line of defence from infection. Alex rushed out to the pharmacy to get it. I hated medication and had refused to take anything other than natural tinctures to speed the labour but nothing to stop the pain. Now I had to take antibiotics. Alex came back and I reluctantly took the pills as directed.

Time was ticking away and I was still only four centimetres when Tara checked and it was nearly 11 p.m. I was worried and exhausted, barely able to keep my eyes open, never expecting to be in labour for nearly thirty-six hours. My time was almost up and my body was fighting a war that it no longer seemed able to win. I didn't want to go to the hospital. I didn't want to give up. I had to try again. But somehow, I knew nothing would change. With more tears falling down my cheeks, I placed my hand on my stomach and spoke to the child I'd successfully carried for thirty-eight weeks and two days. I told my little one that it was time for us to finally meet. That I longed to say hello and see his or her tiny face. To count their fingers and toes. As my child stirred within me, I climbed out of the pool to change. It was time to make the call so that our emergency ride to the hospital could be on his way.

A wave of emotions swelled up inside me, but my job wasn't done. I needed to bring this baby earth side; this happy, healthy and whole baby. So, I pushed my emotions and feelings of failure aside and focused on my vaginal delivery at the hospital.

My emergency contact was late, which was a bit unusual. I found out later that he'd forgotten to put gas in the car and literally had to beg the attendant to fill up his tank. I was just grateful when he finally arrived.

As I got into the waiting car with Alex and Tara in tow, I remember glancing back at our home and thinking it'll never be the same. Little did I know how true that would be.

CHAPTER 8: ADMITTED TO HOSPITAL

"You may not control all the events that happen to you, but you can decide not to be reduced by them."

- Maya Angelou

Early in my life I had an unforgettable experience with the hospital. Admitted at the age of eight with what later became known as Kawasaki's disease, which affects the coronary arteries, lymph nodes and skin, I knew first-hand what hospital staff were like. You either met some really nice ones or those on the opposite end of the spectrum. I learned whom to ask questions and with whom to keep my mouth shut. It was quickly understood that following the rules meant going home early, but not following... well, let's say that wasn't an option for me. The death of my childhood best friend Donna, with her shiny baldhead and gigantic smile the day after Christmas, did nothing but cement the hospital as a place of death in my mind. She was just a child, barely a year older than me. I still miss her.

I opened my eyes, realising I'd dozed off again. It was only the pain of the contractions that kept jarring me out of my sleep. Now was a weird time to remember Donna. Looking around I noticed that we still had a ways to go before we got to the hospital. I prayed all would be well when we arrived. Alex had already called our parents to alert them of our change of plans. By the time we arrived my parents were already outside waiting. Exiting the car took some effort. I leaned on my mum – who was in full mother hen mode – to get inside while Alex checked me in.

We were quickly ushered inside, but my dad and Tara were told to wait outside as only two persons were permitted. No way was my mum giving up her spot to be with me so she and Alex took me in. I was placed in a wheelchair and the orderly was nice enough. For a minute I nearly forgot where I was and all the horror stories I'd heard, but the gloomy coloured walls were a constant reminder.

I can't remember if they put me to lie in the bed first to do a vaginal exam or not, but I do remember that the nurse who examined me was stern and rough. She was plump, with brown skin and hair to match. She would have looked nice enough if only she smiled. Instead she pointed to the bathroom and instructed me to pee in a cup. The bathroom was dull with no seat or paper. I looked around in disgust, not wanting to touch anything, but slowly squatted to pee as she'd asked. When I brought out the sample, another nurse with a voice that grated on my nerves practically shouted, "Why you bring that out for? You should have left it in the bathroom." How was I supposed to know this?

When time came for the vaginal exam, both Alex and my mum were sent out of the room. The plump nurse introduced herself but I didn't care. I just wanted out of this place and to be back home in my bed with Alex holding our baby. It didn't seem like that would be happening anytime soon though, and I was tired of being poked and prodded.

Having reviewed the notes Tara provided, Nurse Plump felt it necessary to lecture me about the dangers of home birth and why I should've come to the hospital sooner. On any other day I would have fought her tooth and nail and reported her to management, but not today. I was tired and everything she said, though unnecessary, was something I'd heard throughout my pregnancy.

I was asked the same questions over and over: how long was I in labour? Why didn't I come in sooner? Was I seriously planning on doing a home birth? The latter seemed to be frowned upon but I didn't care. They had my notes so they could simply read them.

Another lady was being rolled into the room. Her screams sent a chill down my spine. What was wrong with her? It was then I realised this was a public space. There was no real privacy except for the thin curtains that separated the beds. I could hear everything being said and I imagined so could she, not that she noticed anything but the pain. Another scream pierced the air. I wish she'd just stop screaming though. At that moment she turned to her side and I saw her face. I knew her. Suddenly the curtain was closed and her screams stopped abruptly.

I was in another room, but I'm not sure how I got there, or which floor I was on. I just recall opening my eyes and being in a larger room that was practically empty except for one nurse close by the bed and another near the door. The weight on my ankles caused me to look down to see Alex resting on my feet. He looked exhausted, worried and frustrated. It had been a long few days for all of us.

The nurse near the bed came forward. This one at least seemed pleasant enough but, like the rest, she asked Alex to leave the room. I was tired of him being asked to leave. Where was he going? Why couldn't he stay? He was my husband and next of kin. I voiced my concerns and was told simply that it was the standard policy as I was about to have yet another vaginal exam.

Alex explained sometime later that he'd been ushered to the waiting room. At one point while sitting there with his head in his hands, a lady walked past and told him not to worry that everything would be okay.

This vaginal exam offered just as much discomfort as the others, but something was different. When the nurse removed her hand she had a look on her face. Something was wrong. When I asked her about it, she paused for a while before finally saying that she felt hair.

"What do you mean?" I asked.

"Why didn't you tell me your water broke?" she said. "Did it break when you were home?"

Before I could answer, she muttered something I didn't quite understand and walked towards the door. When I shouted after her that I came in with my waters intact and had no idea they'd broken, she didn't even bat an eyelash in my direction.

Alex came back in and I told him what had happened and he was just as shocked as I was. He went to the other nurse at the door and asked when we'd get to see the doctor, but no one seemed able to give a clear answer. We were once again told we'd have to wait.

I lost track of time, each wave of pain bringing me closer and closer to my breaking point. My back was still on fire and both Alex and I were exhausted. He could barely keep his eyes open and was nodding as he stood beside the bed, so I didn't want to bother him to do more compressions. I needed this baby to come out, especially as my hopes of a vaginal delivery were waning.

No one was coming to us, no nurses, no doctors and the pain was getting worse. Although I had taken the antibiotics for the Group B Strep, I was still concerned as the nurse said my water broke and there was still a risk to my baby. I couldn't understand why no one was doing anything and a strange feeling I couldn't shake was building in the pit of my stomach.

Alex had fallen asleep again at the edge of the bed and I had to admit to myself that I wasn't going to have the birth I intended. I signalled the nurse on sentry duty by the door and asked her if there was any way I could see a doctor or get a caesarean section to get my baby out now. She stared at me and just repeated the monotone line: the doctor will be with you soon. But something was definitely wrong and she didn't seem to be listening. I was neither doctor nor nurse but I knew my body. My child was not descending and I wasn't dilating further. I'd been at this since Monday and it was Wednesday morning. Was this normal?

I didn't bring this child all this way to lose him or her now. No. Something had to be done and soon. Even the nurses had whispered among themselves about me still only being four centimetres. My child was apparently stuck and I was slowly feeling like there wasn't much else I could do. I silently prayed, "Lord, don't let me lose this child."

Alex woke up, immediately asking what was wrong when he saw the look on my face. I told him the baby needed to come out now. I couldn't understand why the doctor hadn't come yet, especially seeing as my water broke, according to the nurse who said she felt the hair on the baby's head. I felt helpless and at the mercy of the hospital staff. I managed to glance at the clock on the wall. It was already after three in the morning, three hours since I was checked in.

There was a sudden noise that I didn't quite understand at first. Alex heard it too and asked, "What's that?" I turned to look at him for some kind of reassurance or the calmness that I knew him to maintain even in a storm, but there was none. My heart sank as the reality of what the noise meant started to sink in.

"It's the baby monitor," I said. "The baby's heart rate is dropping."

Neither Alex nor I remained calm; the fear and doubts were clearly evident on both our faces.

There was no need to call a nurse or doctor. Before we even had time to process what the dropping heart rate could mean, the once empty room became a hive of activity. Everyone, who moments before just seemed to be idly sauntering by, was now at full alert. Something was definitely wrong. Nurses, doctors and a bunch of people filled the room, all talking at once, saying things I couldn't understand. No one talked to me directly. Alex disappeared from view, swallowed up by this mob of strange, unfamiliar faces.

I later found out from Alex that he was ushered outside and given an update that they would be taking me to the operating room. A nurse took him down to where I would be and he was instructed to wash his hands, put on a gown, shoe covers and a cover for his head. He was then taken to another room to sit and wait. Little did I know that while I was in one room battling my own fears, he was by himself grappling with his own.

I never liked crowds and avoided them like the plague. I could feel the panic rising inside and fought the urge to scream and push myself off the bed. I was feeling closed in and claustrophobic. It didn't help any when the girl who reminded me of a pixie shoved a clipboard of endless papers in my face for me to sign. Where was Alex? Her mouth was moving but nothing she was saying made sense. She shoved the pen at me and I scribbled something onto the pages, briefly wondering how I could legally sign anything when I was so heavily intoxicated by the pain.

I looked around, still unable to find Alex as I was wheeled quickly into the operating theatre. I knew something was wrong but no one told me what it was. Suddenly the fear of dying on that table became real. I had to shift my thoughts to something else and pray and convince myself that I would not die today. I sourced whatever sanity and stubbornness I could find to remind myself that I was not done yet and declared I would be bringing my baby into this world. Entering the theatre, I began to pray for all to be well, praying harder than I ever had in my entire life.

A guy I could only assume was the anaesthesiologist told me to curve my back so he could insert the medication. Curve my back? I leaned over as best I could, not sure what else he could mean. He said, "No, curve your back like a C." How the heck was I to do that? I was already leaning as far as I could. He muttered something and pushed me down a bit before sticking a large needle into my spine.

CHAPTER 9: THE OPERATING ROOM

"One day, someone is going to hug you so tight that all your broken pieces will stick back together."

- Unknown

I don't recall the exact details of being in that room, but I knew the fear that gripped me as I lay there fighting desperately not to panic. My first encounter wasn't the most pleasant and I hoped the rest of the time would be.

My glasses had to be removed, making me even more nervous and helpless as everything went from clear to blurry blobs of colour. I felt like I was stuck watching a horror movie that I couldn't control, with a sea of people with no faces – no eyes, no mouths, no noses. Just a blob above their necks, speaking a language I didn't understand. I'm minus nine in one eye and minus ten in the other. A fancy way of saying my eyesight is horrible. It was only then it crossed my mind that maybe I should've worn my contacts.

There was still no sign of Alex. Apparently, he was still in the waiting room outside. I found out later that when they came out and handed him my glasses, he started to cry as he wrestled with the possibility that he was about to lose his family. Later, he described the room he was in as cold and lonely, saying he'd been there for a while just waiting to be called in.

I was awake throughout the surgery but it felt like an out-of-body experience. Like a bad indie movie where the woman was being taken advantage of against her will and her once bellowing screams of protest became silent cries as her body surrendered to the abuse.

I felt raw, exposed and opened, with hands pulling and tugging at my insides, invading my privacy and my peace. I was swallowed by an emptiness that could rival the depths of the Grand Canyon. Something was missing and I felt rather than saw when my baby was removed from the only place he or she knew as home.

I don't remember when Alex entered the room, but I was thankful to have him beside me holding my hand. My already blurry vision was clouded with tears as I looked at him and I felt a bit of calm return. Our baby had made it into the world and Alex and I were together. He smiled at me briefly before looking over to where they had taken our child. The baby wasn't crying.

We couldn't see what they were doing, nor hear what anyone was saying and I could feel the panic resurfacing again. Just as I was about to speak, a woman turned and said it's a girl and my child let out a beautiful cry right on cue. She brought this crying pink blur, wrapped in what looked like something green, for us to see. And I wondered where my glasses were as I could barely make out her face. A girl? Is that what the lady said?

I asked her to bring the child closer so I could get a better look. My eyes filled with more tears as I was finally able to make out most of her face. She was perfect. Two eyes, two ears, one little 'cataspanic' nose – a term my brother always used to describe our broad noses – a full head of hair and a cute little mouth. I wanted to touch her and was about to ask to hold her, but the woman quickly moved away, taking her out of the room.

Someone said, "Dad, go with the baby. They're taking her to the NICU – Neonatal Intensive Care Unit." Alex paused to kiss my forehead, and then both my baby and my husband were gone. The sound of the closed door brought home the reality that I was once again alone. I was left there on the table in this brightly lit room, exposed and surrounded by unfamiliar sounds, smells and faces. I felt lonelier than I've ever felt in my entire life. Amazed probably isn't the best choice of words, but I lay in amazement that it took less than five minutes for my family to be scattered.

On the other side of the door, walking quickly down the hall, Alex was following closely behind as they rolled our baby in the cot. When they arrived at the NICU, he was told once again to wait outside for a few minutes. As the nurse came out to tell him he could go in to see the baby, he happened to look outside. The rain had started to fall and he took a picture to show me later. When he got to her cot, he looked at the tiny human laying there and smiled. He looked at her tag, noting her time and her weight, but no name. He took some more pictures to show me and after a few more minutes was told he could go up to see me in recovery.

I longed to be home where it was safe, with Alex and our baby. I didn't even get to tell her her name. Nothing had gone according to plan. I didn't get my home birth and felt robbed of my vaginal delivery. I felt broken as thoughts of failure started encasing my mind and I blamed myself for giving up. Maybe if I'd just fought harder or pushed harder. I wanted to go home. I wanted to be somewhere else, anywhere else but here, bleeding on this table, exposed by the bright lights to these uncaring eyes.

A river of tears ran freely down my cheeks as I cried at the loss of the birth I wanted and for the child who was whisked away. In the midst of it, a calming voice came close to my ear. I couldn't make out her face, but she assured me everything would be okay. Somehow, I believed her.

"They're just closing you up now and your husband has gone downstairs with the baby," she said.

She was a doctor, an intern, and I felt comforted by the fact that she took the time to sit with me and explain what was going on.

"Where are my glasses?" I asked.

She repeated the question throughout the room and soon a response came confirming my glasses were with Alex. So my world of blur would continue a while longer. As they closed, I looked up to stare into the silver reflection of the overhead light, trying my best to understand what was happening to the pink and reddish blurbs of my exposed body. Another tug. And another. To my mind it was painful. To my heart it was yet another blow. Proof of my failure.

I told them I could feel them, feel their hands pulling at me, but they said it was just discomfort, so no one listened. I told myself maybe they were right and just faded into the pain and the solemn song that the strange room played, a song of whispers, machines and my beating heart.

I was in another room, no husband, no baby and more unfamiliar faces passing up and down. Had I fallen asleep?

"Where am I?" I asked to no one in particular and was glad when a voice responded, "You're in recovery."

I still couldn't see much and wondered if I was the only patient in the room. I was near the top by what looked like a door, where everyone could pass and see me. This place offered no privacy. I tried to stay awake so I could be aware of all that was happening, but I was heavily medicated and could feel my eyes drooping again and again. I lost track of time.

The slight rubbing of my fingers awakened me. What was that? I couldn't help but smile when I turned to see Alex standing beside me. He looked tired. Really tired. But he smiled back and I knew everything was okay. He leaned over to kiss me, but I asked instead, "Where are my glasses?" He laughed, reached into his pocket and placed them on my face. I was glad to finally see the world in focus again.

No one had explained why our daughter needed to go to the NICU or how long she needed to stay there. I took the antibiotics, but at the time I wasn't sure of the risks for Group B Strep and was terrified that something was wrong with my little girl.

Alex brought pictures of her to show me and told me how she'd settled in. I was torn. I wanted to see her. I wanted to hold her. But I couldn't. At least not yet. I was to be taken down to the maternity ward and Alex was gathering all my stuff. It felt like I'd been there for days.

On the ward, I was once again placed at the top of the room, near the walkway. I didn't like be so near to all who walked by, but I didn't complain. At least it was near the bathroom and near enough to the nurses' station. Alex had to leave. He called my dad to get a ride home and called Jennifer soon after to let her know the baby had arrived so I wouldn't be back out to work for a bit.

After I settled, a nurse with jet-black hair that stood in contrast to her white uniform came forward to inject something into my IV. As a person who was anti-medication and desperate to regain some level of control over my body and what was happening to me, I naively asked her what it was. I was immediately sorry I asked. Without even looking in my direction she barked, "It's what the doctor prescribed."

CHAPTER 10: WITH OTHER MOTHERS AND THEIR BABIES

"Anyone can give up, it's the easiest thing in the world to do. But to hold it together when everyone else would understand if you fell apart, that's true strength."

- Unknown

I wanted to see my baby, to really see my baby, not a blur or an outline. It was bad enough to have to go through the surgery but now I had to stay in an open room with other mothers and their babies, with rude nurses and random strangers coming in to visit their loved ones. Their eyes always seemed to hold the question, curious to know where my baby was. Or maybe it was my overactive imagination. Thankfully for them, no one dared to ask.

Even when my family came to visit it didn't make me feel better. Don't get me wrong, I was glad to see my mum and dad. It was good to be fussed over for a bit. Even Alex's parents, cousins and a few of my friends popped by. But everyone wanted to see the baby and wanted to know where she was. I knew they meant well, but each time somebody asked where she was, it was a reminder that I barely got to see her. Although grateful, I was hardly pacified by the four images Alex took for me, but they were all I had to hold on to when night fell and both she and Alex were gone.

Nights were particularly hard. Since being married, this was the first time Alex and I wouldn't be sleeping side by side in our bed. I missed him terribly. I also missed our daughter. As the babies in their cots started to cry beside their mothers' beds in need of milk and hugs, I cried too for my husband and for my daughter and longed for morning to come.

The next morning my body felt stiff, like it does the day after strenuous exercise, but way worse. I rubbed my nose to ease the soreness from the imprint my glasses had made. I hadn't removed them last night as I usually do, not because I'd forgotten, but because I was afraid to take them off.

Afraid to be in the maze of blurry faces and colours again.

It was probably close to 6 a.m. and some of the mums were already up and nursing their babies, or changing pampers. I couldn't help but feel sad and empty as I watched them. I reached for my phone to call the only person who could possibly understand what I was going through. At hearing his groggy voice, I knew I'd been right to call. He was now waking up and if he didn't get ready soon, he'd be late for work.

"Hey, A. Did you sleep well?" I asked. He groaned, still feeling the effects of the last few days.

"I'm still in bed. You okay?"

I could hear the concern in his voice, but didn't want to burden him so early in the morning. He had a long day ahead.

"I'm good, just missing you a bit," I said. And we chatted for a few moments before he had to go and get ready. As the call ended, I felt alone again.

A nurse came forward and introduced herself as Nurse Olotte. I liked her immediately. She was tall with fair skin, plenty size and a motherly air. I pictured her giving away many a hug to small children. She was definitely a welcomed breath of fresh air in this otherwise horrid place. She wanted to check my incision and give me my sponge bath. As she examined the wound, I winced and she apologised for the discomfort. She explained that everything looked good, but she needed to give me some medication and it needed to be injected at the incision site. I told her to go ahead and braced myself for the pain.

She left and returned shortly after with a large bowl filled with water and sponge. I removed most of my clothes and Nurse Olotte assisted where necessary with my bath. She kept the conversation light and helped me to towel off and redress, but not before removing the catheter. Funny enough, I had no idea it was there, but it certainly made its presence known when it was removed.

Nurse Olotte explained that although my body may feel a bit sore right now, it was best that I move around soon. This would help with my circulation and ease the stiffness. She also warned that since the catheter was removed, I'd need to take my regular bathroom breaks, but she advised me to take it easy.

Due to the surgery, I was on a 'liquid food only' regime consisting mainly of tea and soup, neither of which were pleasant, but I drank it all to regain my strength. There was nothing for me to do but lie in bed and message whomever was available. It was either that or watch the other mothers and their babies.

I'd fallen asleep and was awakened suddenly by one of those dreams where you're walking to the bathroom. Forgetting for a minute that I wasn't home in my own bed, I was startled by the coldness of the metal bed rail. I tried to swing my feet, but was quickly reminded by the sheer pain that I needed to take my time.

My bed neighbour, Sam, was coming around the corner and asked if I needed any help. I asked her to signal one of the nurses at the nurses' station, but they were having a discussion and asked for me to wait. I should have known. After a few more minutes I started waving, hoping to get the attention of one of them, but they continued talking. My bladder felt like it was about to burst and I could hardly move. I needed to pee and I wanted my shoes from under the bed. No way was I walking barefooted on these floors. I considered just wetting the bed, but figured that would only frustrate the nurses and I'd have to lie in it anyway.

I signalled the nurses again and was relieved when one finally came. I asked her to help me out of the bed and if she could get my shoes. She looked at me like poison, but got the shoes and grabbed my arm to help me sit up before she went on her way. I stood there for a minute still in shock by her poor bedside manner.

"You've got this," I whispered to myself, louder than I thought, as I made my first step towards the corner of the bed. It hurt, but this was necessary for my recovery, as Nurse Olotte had said. Each step was going to bring me one step closer to my child. Gripping the IV, I started the most painful walk I'd ever taken, up the corridor to the bathroom, grateful to be as close as I was to the door.

Squatting and preparing to pee was another challenge. The dull bathroom looked identical to the one I had seen when I first came. At least this one had toilet paper. As I prepared to wipe, I was overwhelmed by the amount of blood. Was that my blood? There was blood on the seat and on the floor. I didn't want to panic and focused instead on getting myself and the stall cleaned up.

After the cleaning I walked over to the sink to wash my hands. I felt exhausted and desperately needed to lie down. I had definitely done more than I should've and was grateful when I finally reached the bed. Sam was there watching me and asked if I was ok. I told her about my caesarean and we exchanged birth stories, interrupted by her daughter's cry for food and attention. I was happy for her, but I wanted to see my baby. Being here with all these other mothers and their babies wasn't making me feel any better. I hated it here. I hated this place. This time I had no strength to fight the battle in my mind that said I had failed. I had failed and found no grace to console myself.

PART 3: THE MOMENTS AFTER

"I don't go by the rulebook; I lead from the heart, not the head."

- Princess Diana

CHAPTER 11: SHOULDN'T IT BE NICER IN THE NICU?

"Courage doesn't always roar. Sometimes courage is the little voice at the end of the day that says I'll try again tomorrow."

- Mary Anne Radmacher

It hurt to walk, to even move. Had twenty-four hours even passed since? I wondered. I never thought I would ever have to say I had major surgery, but yet here I was with a ten-inch incision. I hated it. I hated this cut that would now be with me for the rest of my life. Alex said to think of it as my battle scar, as the scar of a proud warrior, but it was too soon. Maybe it was a battle scar. A battle of life and death, I guess. But it was also a reminder that I failed to bring my baby earth side via a home birth and a vaginal delivery.

A number of articles I'd read online providing a definition of 'real' childbirth came to mind. Many of the articles were describing caesarean birth as the coward's way out, even saying it wasn't real birth. To be honest, I couldn't understand why any woman would volunteer to have this surgery and I still can't, but it's their choice. Now having experienced it myself, there's no way I would ever say this way was the coward's way. The recovery time and the pain were way worse. Birth is birth, whether vaginal or otherwise.

Tired of waiting, I pushed up from the bed and walked what felt like a mile to the nurses' station to ask about the visiting hours for the NICU. I still didn't know why she was in there or how long she had to stay. All I knew was I wanted to see my child. Of the three ladies at the desk, one turned to answer and called down to see if the unit was opened. I wasn't surprised when they weren't. It was already ten thirty and visiting hours were from ten to twelve. My impatience was showing but I didn't care.

I wanted to see my child. The baby I carried for nine months and hadn't even gotten to hold yet, much less see her properly outside of pictures. Each time I thought of someone else holding her, feeding her, or just touching her I got upset. I was supposed to hold her first. I wanted to catch her in the birth pool and draw her out of the water and hold her close to my chest and just gaze at her. But I didn't even get that initial skin-to-skin contact that is so critical for mum and baby right after birth. I was her mummy and I loved her, so the first person doing anything for her should be me.

As the thought settled in my mind, it was still hard to believe. I was a mummy. I walked back to my bed to wait until the NICU was open, my eyes blurred by tears. I was a mummy, willing to do whatever it took to see my child. But I was helpless against the rules of this place. I lay down to gather my strength, determined to see her soon, even if I had to walk three flights of stairs to get there. It was my job to love and protect her as best I could and let her know I was here for her. Now if only these people would just let me see her.

At eleven o'clock, the nurse finally signalled to me that they were ready and an orderly was at the station ready to wheel me down. I barely managed to stop myself from saying that it was about damn time. I sat in the chair, grateful to be off my feet. The orderly was mindful not to jar me suddenly but maintained a brisk pace, which I liked. It was almost as if he understood how badly I wanted to get to my destination.

He brought me right to the door where I had to go through the process of washing my hands before entering the room. I expected to be taken to her immediately, but was told to sit and wait. I was tired of waiting, but took a seat near to another waiting mum. She looked about my age with brown skin and locked hair. I wondered briefly what her story was before my thoughts went back to my little girl. I was looking forward to telling her her name. Would she know me? Would I be able to hold her? How much time would I have? Would I be able to breastfeed her? All these questions ran through my mind as I watched people walking around the room.

I wasn't sure how long I'd been sitting, but it was definitely long enough for the pain of being so upright in the hard chair to take a toll. Still, it was nothing compared to the giant chasm growing in my heart, growing deeper with each minute that passed. I was getting angry. Unable to do much more than sit and watch as who I assumed to be the lady in charge took the time to show some workmen where to install hand sanitiser machines. It was the first time in a long time that I felt the need to curse. My incision was throbbing and I could feel the blood rushing to my temple. I needed to calm down. Tara said I needed to maintain positive energy, especially when meeting my girl for the first time. I took a few deep breaths, trying not to think about the time that was ticking away while I had to sit and wait.

I always imagined the NICU to be a magical place with the nicest nurses, the best doctors and the best overall care. After all, this was the space dedicated to the care of tiny humans. The reality was far from expected. I couldn't take it anymore, and started to get up from the chair just as the lady finally came forward and asked us, me and the girl beside me to follow her. As we walked through the room, my eyes wandered to each cot in search of my little girl. She stopped and I looked down at the tiny human lying there, disappointed that the child was not mine. She started to speak but I couldn't hear anything she was saying as I searched the room again. Where was my child? Where was she?

The room was cold and brighter than the maternity ward, only making me wish for the hundredth time that we were all home. The lady was staring at me, asking me something, but I couldn't say what it was. We stood there for a minute staring at each other but not saying a word and I almost laughed at the slight annoyance on her face. "That's not my child," I said simply. She looked at the chart to confirm what I already knew and mumbled an apology before turning her attention to the other mum. I was left to wait again, constrained by the policies and procedures of this place.

She turned and I followed her, finally able to go to my child. There she was. I could feel the tears swelling up in my eyes as I watched her sleeping peacefully. Before I could pick her up, the lady stepped forward, instructing me to put on a gown first. I reached gingerly for the gown at the bottom shelf of the cot, careful not to jar my stitches. I longed for the skin-to-skin contact so she and I could bond, but rules were rules.

All bundled up she looked so fragile, totally oblivious to the world around her. I was surprised at how scared I now was to even touch her after waiting so long. Eagerly, I reached down to pick up this tiny human who was merely five pounds and thirteen ounces. I held her to my breast and managed to whisper the words I'd been longing to say for so long… "Hello, baby." She stirred as I continued to whisper to her, "Your name is Amaiyah. I'm your mummy. It's nice to finally meet you."

An unmannerly voice broke the wonder of our moment, saying, "If you're holding the baby you need to sit down. Don't stand there holding the baby like that."

I turned in the direction of the voice to see a lady glaring at me from the cot to my right. I wanted to curse her. Who the hell did she think she was? But nothing was going to ruin this for me. I had waited too long to finally meet my child.

I rested Amaiyah down, careful not to move her too much and wake her from her sleep, before turning to grab a high chair from the table. Sitting too low definitely would not help me right now as I could feel the strain of all the movement across my incision. As soon as I sat down, the nurse said, "Not that chair. Use the other one." I stared in the direction of the condescending tone, but painfully walked over to the next chair as she had instructed. I wasn't going to waste any more time getting upset.

Picking Amaiyah up again, I cuddled her, singing songs and giving praises as tears flowed down my face. I stayed until they said it was time for me to leave. I kissed her on her nose and started counting down the hours until I could return to visit her again.

Visiting Amaiyah was my favourite part of the day. I woke up excited and ready to go. I was going twice a day - during lunch by myself and in the evening with Alex when he came to visit after work. I took the stairs each time, making it a bit tough physically, but I was too impatient to wait on an orderly and too cautious of those creaky elevators to do much else.

The doors to the NICU always opened late, but closed on time, never budging to give back the extra time they stole. Mentally it was another struggle in itself, as there was one nurse who seemed out to get me and took pleasure in letting me know it was time to go. One day in particular, Alex and I were talking to Amaiyah. We wanted her to hear our voices as much as possible. It was almost five and I knew that nurse would come soon. It was the first evening that we were all together and I was already emotional.

"Time to go," she said.

"It's not five yet and you opened late," was my reply. She said they were preparing to close and get the children ready, but I begged her to give me a few more minutes. I wasn't ready to leave.

She stood there staring at me for a moment, but I refused to waste any more time staring at her face.

"You could change the pamper," she said finally. Somehow she seemed to think I'd get upset, but I smiled at the privilege and extra time I'd get.

She stepped back a bit, watching as Alex and I fumbled, unsure of what to do. As soon as I reached for the pampers on the shelf of the cot, she stepped forward.

"You have to wash your hands first. You want the child to get sick?" she said. Alex was visibly annoyed at how she spoke. I grabbed his hand and we walked over to the sink, determined not to let anything steal our first real moment together. We washed and dried our hands quickly and changed our little girl's pamper for the first time. I nearly smiled as I stared down at the dark meconium I'd read about, never knowing I'd be so happy to see poop. Glancing at Alex, I laughed as he skinned up his face at the sight.

"We're changing a pamper," I said, barely containing my excitement. He merely handed me the wipes, obviously not enjoying the moment as much as I was. We kissed her goodnight, promising to visit her again tomorrow.

Before heading out the door, I turned back to the nurse to let her know that I'd be coming down early to breastfeed. She didn't respond and I wasn't surprised. I hadn't managed to breastfeed Amaiyah yet and although I understood that they needed to give her formula to sustain her while she was being monitored in the NICU, it was yet another thing that I didn't want. This merely added to the already long list of things that hadn't gone as planned.

I needed to breastfeed. I was eager to at least be able to nurse my child and was looking forward to the opportunity. Plus, Tara urged me to pump so that I could get my milk flowing, bringing to mind the real possibility that I would be unable to if I waited too long. My body was prepared to produce enough milk to feed my child, but if there was no child to feed, eventually my body would stop producing milk. So, I planned to come down early and feed her before they gave her lunch.

Eager to feed her, I woke earlier than usual the next morning. After the disaster of pumping last night and only getting two drops and sore nipples, I really wanted to get Amaiyah to latch to my breast. When visiting hours came I went to her cot, only to be told that she'd been fed a few minutes ago. I was upset and more convinced than ever that these people wanted to sabotage me. I tried not to let it phase me, but it did. Why would they feed her if I had already told them I was coming?

Seeing her looking up at me was the only thing that helped to calm me down. She was here and she was mine and we'd be going home soon. Humming lightly, I removed the safety clip from her cot and the monitor from her toe and rolled her to the nursing room anyway. We needed a moment alone and a good few minutes to bond.

CHAPTER 12: FEELS GOOD TO HAVE YOU NEAR

"If you run you stand a chance of losing, but if you don't run you've already lost."

- Barack Obama

Amaiyah was being discharged from the NICU today. I can't remember the last time I was this excited. I was a rollercoaster of emotions as I sat anxiously waiting for them to bring her up to the ward. Just the thought of her being with me was a joy in itself. Even Sam was getting excited to meet her.

I was still amazed at how well Sam and I got along. We shared stories of our families and our expectations of mummyhood like old school friends. It helped to ease the pain of those lonely days and I smiled now as she nursed her baby. She was really starting to get the hang of it. I hoped I would also be able to get the hang of it soon.

The last two days of walking the stairs twice a day to see Amaiyah taught me a lot about myself. As a Christian, I strongly believe that all things are possible, but as a woman, I often struggled with self-doubt. I understood the importance and truth of the battlefield of the mind and came to terms with how I allowed the fears of others to cloud my judgement and jeopardise the most important journey of my life.

With each step up and down those stairs, I reminded my body of what it could do and willed myself to get stronger. I could've taken the elevator, but I hated those things and the walk allowed me to think and plan for when my girl and I could go home.

She was finally here and, as I gazed down I still could not believe how small she was. Barely five pounds. She was as heavy as my ankle weight. I changed her out of the NICU clothes and for the first time was able to dress my child. I smiled at her, watching her adjust to the new sights and sounds, fussy to just be able to sit with her without worrying about when time would be up.

Her clothes were too big, more suitable for a child twice her size. But she was in her own clothes, clothes her daddy and I had bought for her. Her peaceful sleep didn't last long. Unlike the other babies who had settled into a routine with their mummies, we now had to get into a groove. She didn't really know me yet, and I guess she, too, was feeling helpless with all that was happening. I didn't know what else to do and felt slightly embarrassed, as she was the only baby crying.

Amaiyah just had her pamper changed, but refused to drink any milk. I was tempted to ask the nurse for some formula, but held my ground, determined not to fail at this too. Her cries were bellowing throughout the ward, breaking through the silence of the night. It was almost midnight and everyone else had turned in. I saw the nurse at the station looking in my direction and I willed my daughter to hush.

Breastfeeding was still some strange phenomenon that neither of us had quite figured out yet. She'd grown used to the large nipples on the baby bottle of formula they fed her, so she wasn't quite sure how to latch to my tiny nipples. Feeling at my wit's end from all the crying, I messaged Tara asking guidance on what I should do. She gave me some helpful tips, but they too didn't work.

Tears were rolling down my cheeks and I took some deep breaths to calm myself. Alex tried his best to talk me through, but it was hard to do, as he wasn't near. Tara said Amaiyah could sense my frustration so I mustn't get upset, but I couldn't help it. No matter how I tried to coax her, she just would not nurse. I was also fully aware of the nurse repeatedly glancing in my direction and silently prayed she wouldn't walk our way.

My nipple just could not compete with that of the baby bottle. I started to mentally prepare myself to lose another battle. I didn't have the birth I planned and now it seemed I'd have to settle with giving my child formula instead of breastfeeding her. I rested her down again and reached for the breast pump in one final attempt to get this child some food. She gave me two minutes of peace and quiet, almost as if recognising what I was about to do. Or maybe she just wanted to rest her voice, as in no time at all she started to bawl again. Holding her in one hand, I used the other to pump, hoping I'd manage to get enough in the bottle so she could drink.

The nurse was walking towards me. I desperately hoped she'd just walk on by, but she stopped right beside my bed.

"What's wrong with her?" she asked.

I didn't answer right away, more focused on the task at hand than on wasting time in conversation with her. She was one of the rude ones and I wished she'd just go back to her desk.

"Why she crying?" she asked again.

"She's hungry and I'm getting her milk," I replied without looking up. She sucked her teeth and simply took Amaiyah out of my hand and turned to walk in the direction of her station. I was shocked and upset and immediately jumped up from my sitting position to follow them. However, I had sprung up too quickly and groaned as I felt the effects. I grabbed the bedrail to steady myself and focused on controlling the wave of nausea that came. My incision was throbbing, but I slowly walked towards the other side of the bed, intent on knowing where she'd taken my child. She is my child and this nurse had no right to just take her.

I looked up in time to see her coming back with what looked like a miniature cup in her hand. I reached for Amaiyah when she got near but the nurse simply said, "Go finish pump the milk. The child hungry." I wanted to hate her and maybe in that moment I did, but she was right. I needed to pump. Using the bed rail, I started the painful walk back to the pump.

She looked at me and asked what was wrong. To which I casually replied, "Had a C-section." I had almost two ounces now. I poured it into the cup and reluctantly handed it to the nurse. Amaiyah looked like she took it in one gulp, so I quickly resumed pumping, grateful that my child was finally drinking something, even if it was from the miniature cup.

The compressions of the pump hurt my nipples, but I squeezed anyway, pumping as fast as I could to refill the cup. My only consolation was that Amaiyah was drinking and that was all that held me together as that nurse held my child. Tears burned and threatened to roll down my cheeks, but I held them back. As I watched her there in the nurse's hand, I prayed that tomorrow we'd finally be able to go home.

CHAPTER 13: RETURNING HOME

*"I am lucky that whatever fear I have inside me, my desire to win
is always stronger."*

- Serena Williams

Time was just ticking away and I prayed that today would be the day I could leave this place. It was hard to believe that I'd been here just three days. It felt like months had passed, maybe even years, and I knew I was changed forever. The lessons I learnt here would always be with me.

It was bittersweet as I watched as, one by one, other mothers packed their bags and said their goodbyes. Needless to say, I was anxiously waiting my turn. Each nurse that passed by I asked the same question – "Can I go yet?" Only to hear, "No, not yet." Finally a nurse came to do the usual pressure and temperature checks. As she came to do mine, realising the baby wasn't latching, she squeezed my breast. I was shocked. What the hell?! Somehow she thought she was teaching me something, saying that's what I needed to do to get the milk out to feed the child. But I felt violated. I was so shocked I couldn't even speak. Instead, I merely stared after her as she moved on to the next bed.

I started to message Alex who was installing the car seat and almost cussing as he explained all that was required to do so successfully. He, too, was hoping that today was the day we'd be discharged and jokingly said, "But the house was so peaceful." I didn't want to ruin the moment and decided against telling him about the most recent assault. I'd tell him later.

Thankfully another nurse came to the bed, this time the doctor was with her and gave me the all clear to go. I reached for the phone to call Alex to confirm I could leave, but the doctor continued saying that the baby wasn't discharged as yet. What on earth did that mean? I wasn't leaving my child here. No way was I going home without her. Apparently, she couldn't leave until she managed to breastfeed properly. It didn't make sense.

I had already planned to nurse her for at least two years. Yet another thing people chose to share their opinions about, but I didn't care. I was of the strong opinion that cow's milk is for cows and breast milk is for humans so no matter what, I was sticking to my plan. My child apparently didn't get the memo and refused to latch under the watchful eyes of the doctor. So, I had to wait…again.

It was time for lunch, but I still could not be discharged yet. So, I sat and ate the food I definitely was not going to miss. Sam and I were the only ones that remained, all packed up and ready to go. My girl was dressed in her last remaining outfit, one that Alex and I had picked out during the early days of pregnancy. Like everything else, it was too big. I even had to put a knot in the pants to ensure it didn't fall off and folded the hat so as not to cover her eyes.

I wanted to go, but the doctor insisted that he had to see my child latch. It was good for development and speech he said, but I just wanted to go. One nurse, realising my difficulty, was kind enough to share a great tip of squeezing my nipple to express a few drops of the milk before getting the baby to latch and it worked like a dream. Lazy, just like daddy could be sometimes, she wanted some milk ready and waiting first before she would latch on. Unlike the nurse before her, this one was calm and soothing and didn't see the need to grab my breast. I'd definitely miss the good ones.

Another doctor passed, but this time I recognised the voice. It was the doctor from the operating room, the one who performed my surgery. I thanked him for all he'd done to save my life and my daughter's. He paused before simply responding that he was just doing his job, leaving me stunned as he walked away.

When the first doctor passed back, he was just in time to witness Amaiyah latching and I was grateful that my child was finally starting to cooperate. The papers were signed off and we were free to go. But now I had to wait for Alex to arrive. Twenty minutes later, he entered the ward and took my bag. It would be good to finally leave this place.

They were power washing just beyond the door as we exited the building. I felt a few sprinkles of water and was about to signal Alex that I was going inside when an unmannerly guard came and asked us to move from there. Alex started to explain that we'd just come down to get the car, but the guy was not having it, giving me yet another reason why I was happy to leave. Alex didn't bother to argue. Not wanting me to have to walk too far, he left to bring around the car and I was painfully aware of the stares in my direction. It took me a while to realise they weren't really staring at me, but at the tiny human sleeping on my shoulder. I hoped that no one would come too close to touch her. Seeing the van pull up, I started to head towards the vehicle, but not before a lady I'd never seen before came forward asking if the baby was a boy or a girl. I gave a quick one-word reply before moving out of arm's reach.

On the drive home, I kept glancing at the tiny person in the back seat. The seat was too big and she was kind of slouched in one corner, but still more secure than me holding her in my arms. The ride was quiet, disturbed only by the occasional horn blowing as both Alex and I were lost in our thoughts. Everything had changed. Even as I looked out at the familiar road, it was as if I was seeing it with new eyes and the reality of the uncertainty that lay ahead held both excitement and fear.

The minute Alex pulled into the driveway, memories of the day I left, and how I left, resurfaced. As he unlocked the door to our home, I reached for the tiny sleeping baby from her car seat. When I left three days ago I knew nothing of what a real struggle was. Yes, I had faced hardships before, but none like what I had just experienced. I left uncertain of my future and that of my unborn child and returned now a warrior, with her in my arms and my scars below my waist.

Each step up the stairs was a painful reminder that my wounds were still fresh, my body was still recovering, my heart was broken and my mind was still frail. Suddenly overcome by a wave of emotion, my knees gave way from the weight of the invisible boulder I had been carrying that represented all that I had been through these last few days. Alex caught me before I hit the floor and held me for a moment as I cried. Looking down at that sweet face still sleeping amidst it all, I wondered how it was possible to love someone so much that had only been a part of my life for such a short time?

Alex guided me up the remaining steps. As we reached the top of the stairs, I looked around, appreciating that he'd managed to remove the birth pool. I wasn't ready to see it. We walked hand in hand to the bedroom and placed the still sleeping baby in the bassinet we borrowed from a friend. With my head on his shoulder, we watched her until I, too, finally lay down to get some rest.

Being home again took some getting used to. It wasn't just Alex and I anymore; now we had a baby and she was sure to make her presence known. Those first few weeks were rough and I remember thinking, people always asked us when we were going to have a baby, but no one actually told us how to raise one. With my caesarean still fresh, I couldn't do as much as I was used to and getting in and out of bed was an experience.

Amaiyah initially spent her first few nights sleeping in the bassinet on Alex's side of the bed so he could hand her to me when she needed to be fed. But somehow, Alex wasn't always able to hear this tiny human bawling at the top of her lungs in the wee hours of the morning. Needless to say, that arrangement didn't last too long. I got up one night and moved her to my side of the bed. I didn't mind waking up to feed her as we'd finally found our groove with breastfeeding. Plus, it was important for me to keep moving around so as not to get too stiff. But I made sure to wake Alex for quite a few diaper changes.

Alex wasn't able to get paternity leave, and could only get two weeks of vacation to spend with Amaiyah and me. When he returned to work, I was terrified of it just being this child and me and now understood why maternity leave was called solitary confinement. My mum offered to come over to help but I was still jaded from my hospital experience and wanted to be in my own space. Plus, part of me still blamed her for not supporting me in my original birth plan.

Being a mum took some getting used to, but after a while Amaiyah and I started to figure things out and develop a rhythm. All fears that she wouldn't know me quickly faded as she almost immediately took comfort on my left shoulder, tucking her little face in the space between my neck and collarbone.

During the day, I sang songs and talked to her about her future and enjoyed just watching her sleep. But she was an exhausting treasure indeed. Friends always advised that it would get easier and to make an effort to sleep while the baby sleeps. But there was always so much to do. Bottles to wash. Clothes to wash and I still had client work that was overdue.

The lack of sleep was taking a toll, not just on me, but Alex as well. One night in particular, I opened my eyes to find Alex leaning in a precarious position with baby in arms, only to realise he had fallen asleep while standing. Moving as fast as I could, I reached to take her from his arms. I was grateful to miss an unlucky blow as Alex swung his arms wildly in an attempt to catch her. Other times it was me sitting at the edge of the bed unable to keep my eyes open with Amaiyah in my arms. But each time Alex reached to take her, I held on tighter, only calmed by the sound of his voice assuring me that he was just going to put her in her bassinet so I could rest.

There were many days I'd call Alex at work just to put him on speaker and say, "Talk to your child. She is giving me stress." After hearing daddy's voice she'd settle down and sleep, only to resume her bellowing the minute he was no longer on the phone. It was constant games of guess what the baby wants, until we learnt the different cries for food, diaper change or comfort.

I saved up enough of my vacation and managed to get almost six months away from the office. I knew they were talking, but I didn't care too much. Three months into my leave, Sarah called unexpectedly. It caught me off guard, until she ruined it by saying my vacation was over and it was time to get back to work. Full of anger, I dropped the phone back on the hook. All this time and she hadn't reached out to me prior, and that's all she had to say? Vacation was over? I strode over to the bassinet to watch my little one sleep. I was in no rush to return to that place. Sarah only confirmed that neither she nor anyone else really cared about me there.

As if I didn't already have enough on my plate, all the pumping to build up my freezer stash of breast milk caused me to develop tendonitis. I could barely hold Amaiyah without pain and the simple pleasures I was now getting the chance to enjoy were being snatched away. Starting therapy was necessary to assist with my function and I was thankful that my mother was able to take me while Alex was at work.

For months I had to wear a resting splint day and night. I willed my hand to get better quickly because I would not wear the brace to work. I didn't need any questions added to the ones I already knew would come.

CHAPTER 14: FORGIVENESS AND MOVING ON

*"The truth is, unless you let go, unless you forgive yourself,
unless you forgive the situation, unless you realise that the
situation is over, you cannot move forward."*

- Steve Maraboli

A few years have passed since my daughter was born, but something triggers the memories of the day of her birth. I still cry sometimes, but definitely not as much as I used to. Writing this book made the pain fresh again, vibrant with those feelings of helplessness. But I remind myself to keep moving on and celebrate the victories, large or small. The reality is, nothing I do can change my birth outcome.

I eventually spoke to my parents about some of the things they said or did that hurt me and gave them a glimpse into what my hospital stay was really like. But I know that when they read my story it'll help them to better understand all I'd been through.

My mum just wanted to protect me and keep me safe so the idea of a home birth scared her. But she didn't realise the damage that going to the hospital had done to me physically in terms of the scar and emotionally in terms of the guilt. I know she was still hurt about not being there for the birth and by my refusal of her offer to come and help with the baby when Alex returned to work. But I needed to work through those stages by myself.

All the while, my dad sat with his head in his hands and I told him how upset I was with him for telling me that home births were illegal. He explained that based on the lady's occupation, he only told me because he felt she knew best. As he spoke, I saw the tears shining in his eyes as he realised how what he said had really affected me.

Everything wasn't resolved right away and it has taken many more conversations since. My mum and I have had many honest conversations and we are rebuilding a deeper more meaningful relationship than we ever had before. And my dad has resumed leaving me to my own devices.

I've aligned myself with a non-profit organisation that focuses on educating women about the beauty of birth and providing them with much-needed alternatives so that they can exercise their right to choose. I also use it as a platform to share my story and learn from others like myself. People who hear home birth immediately think doom and gloom and many don't understand that birth trauma is a real issue.

A friend of mine recently described us as a 'grin and bear it' society, but for people like me, not anymore. I want to see change and as such I have to be the change. Many said I could just write a letter to the hospital but to me it required more than just that. One letter could easily be cast aside, lost away in a pile of papers on someone's desk or in the bottom of a drawer somewhere. But a book would hopefully inspire other women to share their stories, remind us that we're not alone and maybe even encourage us to unite our voices for such a worthy cause.

I want to see public forums supported by the government endorsing alternatives for expectant parents and supporting breastfeeding or pumping in the workplace. I want persons to understand that three months is not enough time to bond with a child you carried for nine months, especially not after a caesarean section and most definitely not after birth trauma. And for dads to get their time as well to be with mum and baby. Dads are needed to lend that helping hand and be that anchor that mamma needs as she comes to terms with all her body has been through.

Aside from that, I'm getting back to the basics of the things I love - singing, writing, photography and enjoying the precious moments I have with my family. I still have difficulty when anyone tries to lift Amaiyah out of my arms or suddenly turns a corner and goes out of sight with her. I also can't bear not spending her birthday with her, but I think I'm on my way to recovery and healing.

Alex and I are talking about having another baby and I'm glad he encouraged me to write. I needed to get all these emotions out in the open first before that could happen. I've accepted the fact that home births are not recommended for mums after a caesarean section, at least not here in Barbados. So, I'm exploring my options. Many articles I've read highlight that having a caesarean section once increases the chances of getting another, but that won't be my next story. I won't be cut open again and I believe in the possibility of vaginal births after caesarean sections. I also have a better understanding of the power of the mind and I've made up my mind. No more cuts.

The days when it gets really hard, I stop and write it down or I pray or I look at my daughter and appreciate every day I have with her now because it could have ended another way.

PART 4: THE CONVERSATION

"I'm looking forward to the future, and feeling grateful for the past."

- Mike Rowe

CHAPTER 15: LET'S TALK

"The more people that I meet in my life, the more I realise that everyone has a story. What I find myself wondering is how many of these stories remain unshared? Forgotten? And ultimately lost through time?..."

- Holly Salsman

Becoming a mother has changed my perspective on many things. It's made me a walking contradiction – more patient, but more impatient, happier but more stressed, more confident but more unsure, more resilient but also more emotional. After a while, I knew I needed help. Not that I was crazy or anything, but I needed to talk to others who were in the same place as I was. I needed to talk to other mothers.

I reached out to a few ladies I knew and started a group called Mums Helping Mums. It's a small but powerful group of ladies, each having their own unique birth stories. There are some who had home births and others with hospital births; some with vaginal deliveries and others with caesarean sections. We've had many a journey and we correspond daily about our adventures through motherhood – the joyful, the traumatic and even the mundane. I've invited a few of these special ladies to be part of an open conversation on the topic of birth and motherhood – facing the challenge of juggling it all.

Korena: The reality is that women don't talk about things as much as society seems to think we do. Yeah, we may talk about clothes and shoes, hair and makeup and even places we want to travel, but we never seem to really dig beneath the surface. A few years ago, a friend of mine asked me if I ever have painful periods. After saying no, I was shocked to learn hers had always been painful and she thought this was the norm. Turns out she'd been suffering from endometriosis for years and didn't realise. She, along with the things I've seen or heard since becoming a mother, has inspired my need to create a platform for women to share and to talk openly beyond the surface and dive deeper into more meaningful conversations.

So, let's begin with something easy. I'm tossing this out here to you ladies: What did you do to prepare for pregnancy or motherhood or both?

Isabella: I can't say that I really did much to prepare. But after my OB/GYN suggested I take some birth classes, I decided to go ahead. The coordinator of the sessions explained about labour, breastfeeding, diet and nutrition, exercise, care of the baby, how to pack your bag. It was a really good prep. I also did some prenatal yoga.

Keisha: I watched a tonne of birthing videos and read everything I could find.

Maleah: I changed my eating habits. I cut out most of the refined flour and sugar, started prenatal vitamins and increased my use of whole grains, fruits and vegetables.

Amelia: I changed my eating habits as well. Like Maleah, I used prenatal vitamins but I also lessened my excessive exercise routine. Before I found out I was pregnant, I used to go the gym and do aerobics but when I found out about the pregnancy, I stopped doing the aerobics. I did continue to walk though.

Charlotte: There wasn't anything that I could say that I did differently to prepare. I just maintained what I've always done, positive thinking and placing everything into God's hands.

Korena: What was your birth experience like?

Amelia: I did not have a natural birth. I had an emergency C-section. Obviously I was sedated throughout the operation. When I awakened, I was in excruciating pain and I just wanted to see my baby whom I was yet to meet.

Melissa: I had a hospital birth and my son was also delivered via C-section. I always figured I'd have a C-section. My mother had two, so I was mentally ready to have one. Plus I'd read somewhere that small women with small feet tend to have caesareans. So when they told me I needed to have a C-section, I wasn't surprised.

Korena: I don't think it ever crossed my mind to think that if my mum had a C-section that I'd likely have one too. But my mum and I actually didn't discuss the real details of her births until after Amaiyah was born.

Isabella: Well, like Melissa, I was also expecting to have a C-section. My mum had one and she and I have a few health challenges in common. I knew home birth wasn't an option for me. So, the choice came down to which hospital I would go to the pricey one where my OB/GYN worked or the public one where she didn't. In the end, I chose the one with my OB/GYN and my mother helped me pay for it.

Keisha: Well, I had a home birth with both pregnancies. They were both born in water in the birth pool. I had it planned to a tee. But it was postpartum with my second that was the issue.

Melissa: I went into the hospital the Friday morning and was induced the Friday night. To be induced they had to insert the catheter and the person that did that…let's just say she didn't know what she was doing. After two failed attempts, someone else had to finish it. Next, I had the experience of a mature doctor teaching a younger doctor how to break my water. Needless to say the younger doctor still couldn't get it done after three attempts and the mature doctor had to step in and do it for him. The Sunday, I got an epidural and a C-section. I could feel the tugging but I couldn't feel any pain and I knew when he came out. I heard when he started to cry. They brought him to me to see before they took him to clean him up. I fell asleep and didn't see him again for quite some time. I woke up with my brother standing over me, in an almost pitch-black room.

Maleah: My birth experience was traumatic. My son was born via vaginal delivery in an overseas hospital at twenty-five weeks. He was three months premature and weighed just over a pound.

Charlotte: I had planned home births with my children. All of my births went smoothly and I thank God for that. They were relatively quick, the longest being 7 hours and the shortest being 3 hours. When my major contractions started, we notified the midwife and she advised us to continue monitoring the contractions. Once the timing between them shortened, we called again and she made her way to us. We called two other people that we wanted present at the birth. When the midwife arrived, it was time for her to examine me. By this time, my husband was instructed to start filling the birth pool with water. When I got in the pool, things went quickly. The warm water was exactly what I needed. It was so relaxing. At this point, the midwives and doula simply encouraged me to let my body do what it was created to do. After some intense contractions, pushing and the ring of fire (that burning sensation when the baby's head is crowning), my little person/people arrived! Through it all, I always felt like I was in control of my body.

Korena: So, did you have a clear visual on how you wanted the birth to go?

Isabella: From the birth classes I attended, I knew I could bring in a birth ball to sit on. So, I planned to do that and walk the halls just passing time until I was ready for delivery. Or sitting in the chair listening to music. But then the pain started and the long and short of it was that concept went through the window. My son was in my back. That entire plan to walk around did not happen.

Amelia: I guess I just imagined it to be painful, yet rewarding.

Melissa: I knew I wanted to stay with my original OB. I really liked her disposition. I remember having discussions with her about birthing positions like squatting and she assured me that I could pretty much do what I wanted. But I didn't have insurance and when I saw the price list for her hospital I knew it wasn't something I could afford, so I had to switch over to the public hospital. But I knew that once I went there, I wouldn't have the same liberties.

Keisha: Well, I had a birth plan. I did all my reading and researching and I knew the direction in which I wanted things to go. But my partner's mother died during childbirth, so I had to be careful about pitching the whole home birth thing to him. My sister had one by accident because she didn't know she was pregnant at the time, so she ended up birthing at home. But to be quite honest, that's when I fell in love with the idea. More and more research brought my partner onboard over time.

Maleah: I had a simple visual of a vaginal, hospital birth. My OB works at the public hospital, so there wasn't any need to switch. It never crossed my mind that the hospital would be overseas.

Charlotte: I wanted the delivery to go quickly and be as painless as possible.

Korena: What part would you say was most challenging?

Melissa: I'd have to say the breastfeeding. He wouldn't latch. I actually didn't get him to breastfeed until three days after he was born. All that time he was on a bottle. Thankfully, a retired nurse ended up visiting the ward and came and sat with me. She took the time to show me some techniques that may help. She was a godsend. The other nurses were just like, "He gotta breastfeed or you can't leave here." One morning, I was trying to breastfeed and the child still would not latch. So, I went to ask one of the nurses if I could just get a bottle to feed him because he was hungry. The nurse said, "The child has to breastfeed." I tried to explain to her that he wasn't breastfeeding and asked what I was supposed to do. Was I to let him starve? She quickly said they didn't have any more milk. Frustrated, tired, sad... everything, I called my cousin to bring some milk for me. It was weighing me down mentally that I wasn't able to do something that I thought would just be natural and that I didn't have the support that I thought I would have. Even when I got home, they'd say that I should just give the child the milk. I was drinking malt, fennel tea trying anything I could think of - but the milk just wouldn't come. Then there was one instance where I actually got six ounces of milk and I was feeling fussy because I would usually only get two. I decided to put it in the fridge in an effort to start building up a stash. Sometime later I asked my mother to give the baby the milk for me. Somehow, she didn't put the bottle together properly and the milk spilled. I think that just did me in. Then the second thing that impacted me was when my grandmother died. My son was three months. I had now gotten into a rhythm. But the stress of her death just caused everything to stop and my son just stopped breastfeeding.

Isabella: I know you didn't get to do the kind of reading you wanted to, but the reality is that breastfeeding is hard. And there are a number of reasons why children don't latch. Some children may be tongue-tied for example. People always point blame at the mum if the child doesn't breastfeed but that's not always the case. And it really isn't something that's as simple as we think. But we don't know because, like Korena said, we don't talk about it. Then we're dealing with all these hormones. For me, after I took my son home, I was weepy for a few weeks. I just couldn't stop crying.

Korena: Having smaller nipples also causes an issue with new-borns latching, as well as inverted nipples. Tara took the time to explain this to me when I, too, was having trouble breastfeeding.

Amelia: The pain following the C-section and not being able to eat were the most difficult for me. I was on drips for a few days and, as a result, I got gas. But at the end of it all, I must say, just getting to hold my son for the first time was extremely rewarding.

Keisha: I'd say I had a pretty textbook type of birth. The hardest part with my first child was when I had to get my cervix pushed out of the way. Although I was dilating, my cervix was still in the way. That was painful. By the time I had my second child it was almost the complete opposite. I could not function. He was crying at every turn and so was I. I cried about everything, from hanging out laundry to milk not coming in like before. My hormones were just all over the place.

Charlotte: For me, it was the varying levels of discomfort you go through during pregnancy.

Maleah: The waiting. The uncertainty. Watching him in the incubator and just praying that he'd live to see another day. Although I was able to hold him soon after delivery for a few minutes to take pictures, they had to intubate him and he remained in the incubator for two weeks.

Korena: Would you say your family and birth team were supportive?

Isabella: I definitely have to say yes. I mean, there were one or two small moments when a nurse kept telling me to try and rest and get some sleep between contractions and I couldn't help thinking how the hell she expect me to sleep with this back pain?! But aside from that, when I wanted to give up and was saying to give me a C-section, the midwife called my OB to talk me off the ledge. She really was the one who helped me to hold on. She encouraged me to push and allow my body to do what it was meant to do and reminded me to breathe. So, by the time my OB arrived I was in a better place. But I remember there was a point I thought my back would literally break in half. And then my OB said to hang on, he's coming out soon and within half hour, my son was out.

Keisha: If a midwife was able to talk you down from a caesarean then she's a great midwife.

Isabella: My midwife was a rock star. And I was also able to have my son with me breastfeeding for that first half hour before they took him to get him cleaned up. I had an episiotomy, a vaginal cut during delivery and he was on my chest the whole time while they were stitching me up.

Melissa: Isabella, I wish I had an experience like you did.

Keisha: For the first child, I must say, I was loved and pampered. I felt like I had the support needed But by the time I had my second child it was almost the complete opposite. My grandmother was overseas at the time and my mother just wasn't in the mood to assist. She actually told me she wasn't feeling well, so I took the baby to see her only to find out that she was fine and just didn't feel like coming to my house. With the second baby, she took a very hands-off approach and kept iterating that I had it covered. I couldn't get anyone to help me and my son had allergies, so I really needed the help.

Even when I went back out to work, everyone was commenting on how disorganised I was, but no one seemed to understand just how much help I really needed and that I didn't have it all together.

Korena: So, in essence, having that support, whether from family and friends and even the birth team, is critical to how you feel about your children after?

Melissa: Definitely. My mother and boyfriend were there and very hands-on. I was able to sleep during the day. They did everything I needed them to do and that helped immensely. I must take my hat off to single mums. I had all that support and still I had days when I just couldn't figure out what to do with my child. Single mums are superheroes.

Maleah: Both my family and my medical team were extremely supportive.

Charlotte: Mine were too. I wouldn't change them for anything. I'm so happy that I chose to have midwives and a doula as a part of my birth experience. Kathy and Andrea, my midwives, made me feel confident in my ability to make it through the birth process. Their voices were always reassuring and calm. Jan, the doula, also provided much-needed encouragement during each labour experience. My family was generally supportive, but I don't think I would have paid much attention to those that weren't. My mind was already made up.

Amelia: My team was excellent. The nurses were patient, understanding and very cooperative. My family was also super good throughout. My brothers checked in on me daily, my mum prepared meals and my aunt made sure I took my prenatal vitamins and offered medical advice. She even made sure I was booked in advance in a private room at the hospital and when my water broke, she called ahead to let them know to prepare my room so they expected me on arrival. It was great. My siblings also helped set up the nursery and my husband took time off from work to assist me when I was on leave.

Korena: Is there anything you wish you had done differently?

Amelia: I wish that I had exercised more in the early stages because I really wasn't happy with the weight gain, but I had to take it easy as I had a miscarriage just prior to this pregnancy.

Melissa: I wish I'd done some more reading, especially on breastfeeding. Now looking back on it, I realise that nine months is not enough time to really prepare. I also would have gone to the other hospital and stayed with my original OB. I feel like my overall experience would have been better. I probably wouldn't have needed an anaesthesiologist. I probably wouldn't have needed a C-section. But who knows?

Maleah: I don't think there's anything I could've done differently. I think I did the best I could, given the circumstances, and there was nothing that could have prevented my son's birth from happening the way it did.

Charlotte: I would have recorded at least one of my home births.

Korena: Did you always want to be a mum?

Amelia: Yes. I always wanted to be a mum. I absolutely love children and I knew I would be super great at it. I think it's absolutely rewarding and I was happy to spread the love. Now that I am a mother, I must say that it is challenging at times but I love it. It's wonderful.

Melissa: I've never really thought about it one way or the next. I just figured it'd happen when it happens. I never wanted to or not to. I'd been in a relationship for a very long time and my boyfriend and I weren't being that responsible sexually, so I figured if it didn't happen in a couple years I'd have to look into in vitro or something. Then one day he and I had sex and I just knew by the next morning that I was pregnant. When pregnancy was confirmed, I got doubts about it and considered getting an abortion. But after seeing the pain a friend of mine went through after she had one, I knew that wasn't for me and I wouldn't be able to handle that. My relationship wasn't on the best path and we weren't seeing eye to eye, so I didn't know if it was the best time to add another person to this thing, and I wondered how's this going to work. So, I say all of that to say, I don't know. I just expected it would happen. Society tells women they're going to be mothers. It was really only after I had a child that I wondered what my life would really be like now if I didn't have one.

Isabella: I think I've always known I wanted to be a mother. The mother instinct has always been there and I've always leaned more towards the smaller kids. Being raised in the church, I always figured that I'd get married and have a child. But I had a backup plan. I didn't believe that I needed to have a husband to be a mother, even though that may be the traditional way of thinking. I made up my mind that if by age thirty-five and I wasn't in a steady relationship, but felt I was able to afford a child and that I was ready, I was more than willing to ask a friend a question and have the child I wanted. Whether he wanted to be just the sperm donor or he actually wanted to be a father was up to him.

Melissa: I actually saw a video on Facebook about a woman who did just that. And I think that's great. Why should you have to be in a relationship to have a baby?

Isabella: Let's be real. Fertility options are expensive, so if you can find somebody that you know, that you respect, you don't have to be in love with them. Then, why not? A lot of people can't see that but, for me, that was my backup plan.

Keisha: Well for me, the answer is a solid no. I never wanted to be a mother. I never wanted children. I never wanted to be married. My mother reminds me of it anytime I start to complain about the children or my husband. I wanted to build businesses, to travel the world and take my mother on extravagant excursions and do big things. That was my dream. I was gonna be a boss bitch, rolling up in my big-up Jeep and well-educated. I was going to be that aunty and when my sister got children we'd be balling. Now I have two children and I just feel like I'm going further and further down the rabbit hole. If I had to do things over again, I wouldn't have children.

Korena: Wow Keisha. I definitely wasn't expecting that.

Maleah: I've always wanted to be a mum. Before I had my son, I wanted to have five children, but knowing what I know now…that number has been reduced to three. I mean, sometimes being a mother can be overwhelming and really not go according to plan, but then I realise that each day with him really is a gift. So, I try to focus on that.

Korena: I wanted to have six. Maybe I still do, but time and finances will tell.

Charlotte: I've always wanted to have children. It was awesome and empowering to know that I endured the pain and this was my reward! It's great when you realise that you're now holding the little person that was moving around inside of you. New babies smell niiiiice! I love the baby phase (probably why I kept having them). The challenge comes as they become more active. I love their energy, in small doses. I love to watch them sleep, that's the most glorious time of the day. My new normal is tired and I'm learning to accept that.

Korena: Thank you ladies, for taking the time to share your stories. I learnt a lot and I hope that each of you did as well. Maybe someday soon we'd be able to continue this conversation and even turn it into an official forum for mums to share.

PART 5: THE END

*"There are two great days in a person's life - the day we are
born and the day we discover why."*

- William Barclay

CHAPTER 16: AND THAT'S MY STORY

*"Sometimes the strongest people in the morning are the people
who cried all night."*

- Sai Gautam

Looking back on everything now, I am grateful for all that happened. Not that I wanted things to happen the way they did, but I'm glad I made it through. It made me stronger and hopefully my story will now be able to inspire others.

Each day that I'm alive I can't be anything other than grateful. I still have a few down days, a few 'why me' days. But I'm still grateful. Each day with Alex and our daughter is a privilege even if not always a pleasure dealing with the temper tantrums of the terrific twos.

I hope those that take the time to read my story can learn something from it. To the mums-to-be, I encourage you to make the best decision for you, no matter what anyone else thinks. For the dads-to-be, I encourage you to support her, love her and to be there for her. She's growing a tiny human that will be carrying on your legacy someday. To the grandmothers, understand this is not your story, but it's a continuation of your daughter's. She needs you to tell her everything will be all right. Save the horror stories. Save the criticism and just be the best mum you can be to your daughter as she gets the chance to walk in your shoes on her journeys to being a mum herself.

To those in the healthcare industry, know that you matter. To the nurses, midwives, doulas and doctors, see that birthing mother as more than just another patient. She's someone's wife, someone's daughter, someone's sister, someone's friend and she's about to be someone's mother. Cherish them for the work they're doing, helping to bring new life into this world. They're champions. Treat them with respect. They're human. Show them love. Treat them as well as you'd want someone to treat you.

No two births are the same and no two women are the same, but each mum needs love and support during this time. It doesn't matter how old she is or how many children she may have had prior.

Child birth is scary, it's exciting and it's beautiful. But too often it is tainted by lack of support, fear and uncertainty. A negative birth experience is often the reason behind some women not wanting to go through it again. Let's highlight the beauty of it, the joy of it and the love of it and provide woman with their right to choose.

To all mums, I'm proud of you, and even though I may not know you, I love you and I respect you. May we continue to encourage each other. Let's share our stories and let us continue to have the conversation.

ACKNOWLEDGEMENTS

This book was inspired by a curveball of events that happened that I didn't expect. I think it was God's way of propelling me to finally take up the mantle He'd given me of being a writer. And because of all that happened with my birth, I finally did.

God also led me to Donna Every, whom I'd interacted with many times before and I took her writer's workshop. She encouraged me to share my story and willingly shared her knowledge of writing and getting started. Even after the workshop was complete, she still made herself available, at any time of day to answer the many questions I shamelessly bombarded her with.

Thank you to my editors, Toni Daniel and Julia Thorington, for their time, hard work, commitment and dedication throughout this process. Toni, especially, helped to draw out the vulnerability necessary to craft my story on these pages.

Thanks to my dad for always believing there was a writer inside me, and for putting in his special request for another book. Thanks to my mum for reading my story, loving my story and encouraging me to share it with the world.

Special thanks to all the powerful mums of the support group, especially those that took the time to have the conversation with me.

I've already dedicated this book to my husband Alex and my daughter Amaiyah, but I think Alex has earned extra special mention. I'm so grateful to Alex for taking the time to read through my many drafts of this book. He shared his ideas and encouraged me every step along the way. He motivated me during those moments when I wanted to give up. He was my sounding board and the one who got me to open up and be vulnerable in sharing my emotions. When I struggled to write he reminded me it was okay to take a break and he held me accountable to meeting my personal writing schedule. He even set up a dedicated writing space for me and constantly reminded me that this book was the first of many.

Thanks also to those who took the time to review my manuscript and shared your honest feedback.

Finally, thanks to all of you who took the time to purchase this book and share it with others, I will forever be grateful to you all.